WHAT PATIENTS TEACH

WHAT PATIENTS TEACH

The Everyday Ethics of Health Care

Larry R. Churchill

Joseph B. Fanning

AND

David Schenck

OXFORD
UNIVERSITY PRESS

OXFORD
UNIVERSITY PRESS

Oxford University Press is a department of the University of Oxford.
It furthers the University's objective of excellence in research, scholarship,
and education by publishing worldwide.

Oxford   New York

Auckland   Cape Town   Dar es Salaam   Hong Kong   Karachi
Kuala Lumpur   Madrid   Melbourne   Mexico City   Nairobi
New Delhi   Shanghai   Taipei   Toronto

With offices in

Argentina   Austria   Brazil   Chile   Czech Republic   France   Greece
Guatemala   Hungary   Italy   Japan   Poland   Portugal   Singapore
South Korea   Switzerland   Thailand   Turkey   Ukraine   Vietnam

Oxford is a registered trademark of Oxford University Press
in the UK and certain other countries.

Published in the United States of America by
Oxford University Press
198 Madison Avenue, New York, NY 10016

© Oxford University Press 2013

Library of Congress Cataloging-in-Publication Data
Churchill, Larry R., 1945– author.
What patients teach: the everyday ethics of health care / Larry R. Churchill,
Joseph B. Fanning, and David Schenck.
p.; cm.
Includes bibliographical references.
ISBN 978–0–19–933118–5 (hardcover: alk. paper)
I. Fanning, Joseph B., author.   II. Schenck, David, author.   III. Title.
[DNLM: 1. Ethics, Clinical.   2. Delivery of Health Care—ethics.
3. Patients—psychology.   4. Sick Role—ethics.
WB 60]
R724
174.2'8—dc23   2013006810

3 5 7 9 8 6 4 2
Printed in the United States of America
on acid-free paper

Larry Churchill dedicates this book to
Betty Jo Woomer and John Hugh Churchill
siblings, and sages in life's journey

Joseph B. Fanning dedicates this book to
Buck Breland, friend and healer

David Schenck dedicates this book to
Dolly and David, where it all began

The particular beauty of *human* excellence just *is* its vulnerability.

Martha Nussbaum, *The Fragility of Goodness*, 2, interpreting Pindar's *Nemean*

CONTENTS

ACKNOWLEDGMENTS

Collectively, we are grateful to the following people who in various ways contributed to this book: Roy O. Elam, medical director for the Vanderbilt Center for Integrative Health, for the financial support he helped us secure to do this study, and for his encouragement and support as we proceeded; Peter Ohlin at Oxford University Press, and his most able associate, Lucy Randall, who made everything about the process work smoothly; Katie Haywood, for extraordinary skill in formatting and otherwise preparing the manuscript—no one could hope for more competent help; Jessica Ryan, for a superb job of copy-editing the final version of the manuscript; Kathryn Montgomery, who saw our purpose from the beginning, as she did with our previous book, *Healers*, and for her careful readings of both our prospectus and the more polished version of this book; Howard Brody, for his astute comments on the manuscript at a critical stage; Allison Adams, for her as ever incisive and forthright editorial work; Juan-Carlos Monguilod, medical director, and other administrative staff at Hospice and Palliative Care of Greensboro, North Carolina (HPCG), for their invaluable assistance with the 14 interviews with hospice patients. A special thanks is owed to the superb social work staff at HPCG who spoke with patients and families to explain the study and to secure their consent to participate: Holly Bessey, Anne Batten, Debbie Garner, Beth Mills, and Madara Shillinglaw.

Thank you to the clinicians we interviewed for *Healers*, who subsequently provided names of patients for us to contact for these interviews; Ruel Tyson, whose teaching on the richness and wisdom of ordinary practices has been a benchmark for us for decades; to the community of scholars and teachers housed within the Center for Biomedical Ethics and Society at Vanderbilt University, and especially the center's director, Keith Meador; our colleague Paula DeWitt for her assistance with indexing; and our most able and cheerful assistant Denise Lillard, who keeps us smiling.

Our greatest debt and gratitude is to those who consented to these interviews, and to their families who often assisted with the logistics of the interviews. If we have captured a fraction of their insights we will be satisfied.

Larry Churchill thanks his coauthors Joe and David for the fun and the learning that emerged in this project; and his family, near and far, living and dead, whose lives continue to humble and inspire him, and especially—as always—Sande.

Joseph Fanning thanks his coauthors Larry and David for mentorship grounded in mutuality and for book meetings filled with laughter, rigor, and wonder; his parents, Tom and Gail Fanning, for their steady encouragement; his children—Ben, Mia, and Willa—for welcoming him home every night with hugs; and Carrie for her curiosity and companionship.

David Schenck thanks Dick Zaner for opening his eyes to the possibilities for phenomenology and bioethics to enrich one another; Kelia Culley, who has listened again and again to story after story; and his coauthors, Larry and Joe, for making real that conviviality Polanyi says is essential for deep inquiry.

INTRODUCTION

What Patients Teach seeks to answer a fundamental but largely unexplored question: What do patients see as the core elements in forming therapeutic relationships with their healthcare providers? This query leads to a set of correlative ones: What clinician traits are conducive to establishing healing relationships and what are the barriers to such relationships?; How do clinician-patient interactions figure into the larger life of patients outside the clinical setting?; and, When we listen carefully to patients, what are the lessons for medical ethics and bioethics? This volume is intended to serve as a systematic and detailed response to these questions.

We begin with a small segment from one of our first patient interviews. This extract provides a flavor of the kind of interviews we describe and interpret throughout the book. This patient had been seen by multiple physicians and was taking a large number of medications, many in high doses. He was given a diagnosis of ALS (amyotrophic lateral sclerosis, Lou Gehrig's disease). Following this diagnosis he was alarmed and bewildered, and he sought help from a different physician. The passage below begins as the patient recounts his first meeting with the new clinician.

I was shocked. I sat there and looked at him [the doctor] and he looked at me, and he said, "You know you really could have ALS...but you might not. Looking at all these medicines...it could be the cumulative side effects." And then he looked at me and said, "Has anyone ever talked to you about your weight?" And I almost immediately wanted to turn him off. Then this doctor said, "You're on so much medication that nobody's going to want to touch you unless you're in a supervised weight loss program."

The patient's narrative continues:

I was interested, but also irritated. "Please don't give me another speech about my eating." But he talked to me about *me* and about *my life*. I was at that time in the midst of huge conflicts, certainly sublimating my emotions in food—and there was the loneliness...and this doctor was the only one who cared to ask.

Within a few weeks the patient entered into an intensive weight loss program and was able to go off most of his medications and reduce the dosage of the drugs he continued to take. The ALS diagnosis went away. The patient concludes:

He wanted to see all of me. He didn't want to just look at the lab slips. Listen, every time I see the guy I can hug him and tell him everything....I mean he really saved my life. He was to me the real physician.

DISTINCTIVE FEATURES

We believe there are four distinctive features of this volume. The first is the empirical grounding in patient interviews for our interpretations and conclusions. The second is an understanding of illness, and the fragility of life it symbolizes, as central to the human predicament, rather than an occasional aberration. The third is the articulation of an everyday relational dynamic as fundamental to healthcare ethics, displacing the conventional and dominant "big decisions" model. Finally, we are offering here a detailed description of the moral structure and rhythm of these routine clinical encounters, centered in vulnerability and responsiveness—as understood by patients. In short, we reject the assumption that the core values of healthcare ethics have already been named and adequately analyzed by bioethicists and healthcare professionals. Our aim is to provide a more adequate account.

The title of this book describes both its content and its central argument. "What Patients Teach" accurately denotes a detailed description of what patients have told us about how they perceive their relationships with their clinicians, and especially how these relationships become therapeutically significant—a healing factor added to the clinician's considerable technical expertise and pharmaceutical and surgical resources. In addition, the subtitle, "The Everyday Ethics of Health Care," signals that these are fundamentally moral concerns, and that they happen routinely. While regrettably these mundane, moral dimensions are not always recognized, they are not things that arise only when there are big issues or major ethical decisions in play. They are not simply the province of high-drama and high-stakes scenarios, such as in intensive care units when life support is withdrawn or in transplant programs when organs are scarce. The therapeutic possibilities in patient-clinician relationships are inevitably a part of even the most pedestrian clinical encounters, and their moral features—while sometimes tacit and unspoken—are never absent. It is the ethics of who we are and what we are doing when no big decision is at hand. For better and for worse, the quality of those encounters is the conduit through which everything else flows, as the interview segment quoted above powerfully illustrates. The moral quality of these relationships sets the context for all the other more obviously ethical issues that may arise.

OUR MOTIVATION IN DOING THE RESEARCH

We are faculty members at a large academic medical center and our teaching, research, and service is routinely focused on ethics in a clinical context. As part of a clinical ethics consultation service we are called on to confer, advise, and otherwise be available as resources for a wide range of situations. This work brings us face-to-face with many of the most challenging situations patients and their families ever encounter. Consulting on such cases, we have often found ourselves asking how this situation might have gone better. And more generally what would end-of-life care and hospital care in general look like if we truly listened to and attended to what patients and families needed in the healing process. Would the trust between the family and the healthcare team be less damaged if more sustained attention had been given to developing a partnership? Would "difficult" families have been less difficult if a candid prognosis had been given sooner? Could an adversary have been an advocate if there had been greater continuity of providers? Also, like others who work in this field, we reflected once again on how seldom the standard principles of academic bioethics come into play as we work with patients, families, and medical teams. The moral features of the problems we encounter are frequently not addressed in a helpful way when seen as problems of "respect for autonomy," "beneficence," "nonmaleficence," and "justice." Rather they are best understood as breakdowns of trust, absence of sufficient attention to patient or family values, failures to connect on treatment plans, and other misfires of timing or coordination, often lumped together as issues of "communication." Of course there are times when important questions of autonomy arise, for example, in surrogate decision making for severely ill patients. But most often the issues are more fine-grained and more fruitfully probed using other moral tools. The most common problems are best described as misfits or misfires in attitudes, demeanors, aims, goals, and purposes among the players in the complex web of interactions that typify modern healthcare delivery in hospitals.

And this appears to us to be true for outpatient visits as well as hospital-based care. Hence, a large part of our motivation is to seek opportunities to listen carefully to patients and, after conversations with them, to find better ethical concepts and tools for addressing these routine relational issues.

We conceived this volume as a sequel and companion volume to David Schenck and Larry Churchill's 2012 book, *Healers: Extraordinary Clinicians at Work*.[1] *Healers* describes and explores the findings from 50 clinician interviews, probing what practitioners see as the key elements in creating relationships with patients that have therapeutic value. With the valuable addition of our colleague Joseph Fanning, this book moves to the other side of this dyadic partnership and reports on patient perspectives.[2] We believe it is relevant to anyone who routinely interacts with patients in a professional helping capacity: nurses and physicians, health coaches and counselors of various sorts, chaplains, clinical social workers, consulting bioethicists, and many others.

METHOD AND PRESENTATION

To conduct the research for this new volume we asked a dozen of the clinicians described in *Healers* to provide us access to four to six patients to get their side of the story. As with the provider informants, our patient sampling is purposive, focusing on patients who are reflective and articulate, patients who have had many encounters with clinicians for various interventions, and patients who have insight into what works and what doesn't. The resulting 1,600-plus pages of transcripts from these interviews form the basis of this book. Our patient informants span a broad spectrum of conditions—cancer, diabetes, arthritis, metabolic syndrome, heart failure, depression, among others—and with an age range from 22 to 90. We interviewed 35 female and 23 male patients; 51 are Caucasian, 7 are African American.[3] At the time of their interviews 14 of our participants were enrolled in a hospice program. We provide more details about our methods and assumptions in the appendix.

In writing this book we were guided by a basic conviction: We need to let the patients speak in their own words. Primarily this is because the exact formulations of their responses are so often insightful. But it is also the case that their words have a ring of authenticity, a tone of genuineness that paraphrasing cannot capture. Our editing has been modest. We occasionally delete repetition of phrases, the sequences of starting, stopping, and restarting on a subject, and some of the elliptical features of unrehearsed conversations. But we left in place some grammatical gaffes, colloquialisms, and idiosyncrasies as reminders of the common dynamics of conversation, as well as of the individuality of the interviewees who contributed so much to our work. While we are seeking to let these patients speak for themselves, we acknowledge that our interpretive fingerprints are present at every point. The processes of selection, presentation, emphasis, and especially the lessons we draw are our work. While we have sought to interrogate the interviews fairly and thoroughly and present our interpretations with care, we also recognize that other interpretations are possible. There are multiple truths to be discerned. We hope others will be motivated to take up this interpretative task.

CONTENTS

Chapter 1, "Being a Patient and Living a Life," introduces the major themes of the book by way of 10 vignettes or scenes drawn from a single interview. These themes, such as immediate recognition, information flow, human bond, and going the extra mile, represent some of the most frequent motifs from the 55 interviews. These vignettes provide a mapping of a clinical relationship across time. This mapping is important because there is much to learn from the times in our lives when we are patients. Rather than being an interruption or deviation simply to be overcome and set aside when we are well, illness experiences are uniquely instructive about a fundamental dimension of our lives—our human vulnerability.

Chapter 2, "Clinical Space and Traits of Healing," summarizes and illustrates those relational skills and demeanors that enable trust and healing to grow and flourish. Chapter 3, "False Starts and Frequent Failures," is a recounting of the most prominent ways that patients experience relationship failures, sometimes from the initial clinical encounter.

Chapter 4 provides a narration of three of the most trenchant and moving interviews we were privileged to participate in, with short introductions to each and only minimal commentary and analysis. Here we have let patients tell their stories in longer stretches, guided only by the interviewer's questions and follow-up. "Ibuprofen and Love" is about chronic pain and how it is managed. "Staying Tuned Up" presents an alternative model for wellness and for relating to a clinician, and "We All Want the Same Things" is a narrative of healing at life's close.

The final two chapters are an ethical analysis of the findings from our interviews. Here we argue that the structure, rhythm, and horizon of routine patient care indicate the need for a different set of core concepts for understanding and judging the ethics of health care. Both professional expressions of medical ethics and the work of bioethics need to be informed and reformed by this distinctive set of concepts. Providing patient-centered care means taking more seriously patients' moral framing for this interaction.

[1]

BEING A PATIENT AND
LIVING A LIFE

Being a patient is a unique interpersonal and moral experience. Our aim in this book is to map that experience in terms of its *structure*, *rhythm*, and *horizon*. Our claim is that this defining structure, rhythm, and horizon of being a patient is a special window into the most profound dimensions of human life. This claim is not an obvious one and perhaps not an easy one to entertain. Most of us are routinely focused on health and wellness as the normative state, and as such we tend to overlook or discount the insights available from periods when we are less than well. Health tends to be the norm, if only in our aspirations, for both our sense of self and our moral framework. Contrary to this tendency, we argue that what we can learn from being a patient, from its interpersonal dynamics and its moral contours, is especially instructive for how we experience our lives. Our aim is to open that instruction book. In so doing we focus not on the experiences of illness so much as the experiences of seeking help and building relationships that can be healing. There are many excellent accounts of illness and its meaning.[1] There is little about how healing relationships are formed, why they succeed or fail, and how these relationships come to disclose basic truths about our lives, and especially about our moral self-understanding. This effort is one of probing and elucidating just what the patient interviews offer us as we try to understand—not just in our heads, but in the living tempo of our lives—what it means to be human.

Our task here is one of providing a response to this question: What new possibilities for being human can we discover if we listen carefully and deeply enough to what patients have to teach us? Or, alternatively: What can we learn about living every day of our lives from the times in our lives when we are patients?

During many of life's major crises one is a patient, or someone close to us is one. During these crises, a critical point is made: The vulnerability of life itself, of our very lives, is what leads us to become patients. Becoming a patient is not a matter of being a failure at living; becoming a patient is a direct and indeed expected condition of being vulnerable. And vulnerability is itself a condition of, even a definition of, living. Being a patient thus should not be thought of as a pathological state. That being the case, it follows that clinicians and healthcare professionals can claim no monopoly on interpreting the meaning or the significance of being a patient. This is especially so when it comes to addressing the moral significance of what the patient undergoes during the course of an illness.

The reality of the vulnerability of living is a thread running through all our interviews. Over the last three years we have listened to our interviewees talk about where their lives have been broken, and where they have been healed. Both of these are parts of being vulnerable. We move within seas of bacteria that make living possible—make all of life possible, not just ours. Yet, depending on bacteria as we do, we are vulnerable when they turn on us. We are, that is, fundamentally intertwined on every conceivable level, in ways we do not usually consider, with the world we live in, such that it is often impossible to make a distinction or find a boundary. And wherever we are intertwined, we are vulnerable, we are at risk. We are vulnerable to a myriad of disruptions of this intertwining. Likewise, however, we can grow and learn and we can heal and recover wherever we are intertwined. This is what it is to be human, to live, to exist. There is no easy separation of body and world—and no easy separation of body and self. Indeed, it is most often when we find a gap between our bodies and our selves, our bodies and our world, that we become patients. It is then that we seek to establish relationships with practitioners to aid us in addressing these lacunae and disruptions. And it is out of this possibility for coming apart, out of experiences of the rupture of what binds us to what we most care about and live for, that we become patients.[2]

To get to a place where we can see this clearly, we need to make a distinction between being ill and being a patient. From there, we will sketch out varieties of vulnerabilities in life that impel people to seek healthcare practitioners and become patients. We will then examine common vignettes of clinical life taken from our interviews and in so doing begin a mapping of the experience of being a patient. That work will prepare us for the more detailed analysis of the interviews in the chapters that follow.

DISTINCTION: PATIENT AND ILLNESS

In one way, the distinction between being a patient and being ill is very simple. Being a patient simply means being in relationship with a practitioner. Of course, one can be ill and still not be a patient. And some patients are quite healthy. But things can get rapidly more complex: You can be ill and decide not to go to a practitioner and become a patient—maybe because your illness seems to you to be slight and your likelihood of recovery great. Or, on the other hand, because you are quite severely ill, you anticipate that only additional pain and suffering will result from becoming a patient. Or maybe it is because, even though you are ill and want to see a clinician, you cannot—because there isn't enough money, because there are no practitioners you can get to, because your family will not allow you to go to the practitioner you think you need to see.

Most fundamentally, being a patient entails having a relationship with a clinician—whether short-term or long-term—that is defined by a shared intention of caring for the health of the patient. This relationship is established when both parties are aware of and focused on the threat or reality of illness for the patient. And, likewise, the threat or reality of pain and suffering. Finally, whether working on wellness, an infection, or a life-threatening tumor, the relationship between clinician and patient always takes place within the horizon of death—whether that is near or far, feared or accepted. These elements are summarized in Table 1.1.

Note that we do not need—nor do we wish to use—languages of disease to depict the condition of being a patient. It is an unfortunate narrowing of the moral scope, as well as of the nature of healing, to reduce being a patient to a matter of "contracting a disease," "suffering from a condition," or "having an accident." All these may name experiences a patient undergoes, but they do not delimit or define what it is to be a patient. Disease taxonomies are potent, efficacious abstractions. These abstract disease labels therefore readily become systems of "not-seeing." Not-seeing illness. Not-seeing people. Not-seeing patients. Classifications of diseases of course have their uses, but they are more limited in scope than we commonly recognize. It is seldom remembered that the potency of these classifications can render them toxic.

We want as much as possible to resist the language of pathology and pathologizing that is built into our everyday usage and is so characteristic of talk about patients, especially within medical communities. At the same time, we want to avoid substituting technical or pseudotechnical vocabularies here that result in neologisms like "patient-hood." We go back to the simplest formation: Being a patient means being in a relationship with a practitioner.

Table 1.1 BEING A PATIENT

Being a patient involves:
- Relationship with a clinician
- Shared intention to care for the health of the patient
- Threat or reality of illness
- Threat or reality of significant pain/suffering
- The horizon of death (near or far)

DECIDING TO BECOME A PATIENT

Becoming a patient entails entering into a very specific kind of relationship, with very important consequences for oneself and one's life, as well as one's social world.[3] How and why our interviewees made this most significant decision was of great interest to us. As noted earlier, one of the first questions we asked patients was: How did you decide to make your first visit to him or her? What was going on in your life at that time?

In turn, what do we learn as we attend to the answers patients gave to those questions? Sometimes we go to a clinician because the body just isn't functioning as we think it should:

> I wasn't really sick, but I'd had some issues with blood pressure and I just felt like I wanted to experience acupuncture. I'd heard about it and I was just really drawn to it. I wasn't really, like I said, sick or having a lot of medical problems and we just established a relationship. So I started seeing her once a month, but for me it's been mostly just preventive medicine, just whatever's going on for that month that might be out of balance.

But sometimes the dysfunction is sudden and dramatic:

> I was going around to the car to open the door, and all of a sudden I was looking up at him. I was on the pavement, and I thought, "Good gosh, what a feeling," I wasn't dizzy or anything, just, you're just gone. But I came right back—opened my eye, and there he was looking down at me.

And often enough there is a significant amount of pain accompanied by the body's malfunctioning:

> I thought I had a stomach ache, stayed home a day, kept hurting, stayed home another day, and I just had a bad stomach; she says, "You better go to the doctor, you better go see about that.

You better go to the hospital, something." I said, "Well, okay."
So, I went over there, and they operated on me that night. They
thought I had a hot appendix.

And then there are those events that seem to come from nowhere.
Explaining how he came to be seeing a urologist, one patient
explained, "Well, I went to him when I was diagnosed with a lump
on my prostate." The arrival of this diagnosis coming as directly into
his life as his words came into the interview. Here is your new world,
ready or not.

And then there is that distressing and so often embarrassing element of our vulnerability: The sense we sometimes get that some
part of our body, some aspect of ourselves has turned against "the
rest of us." Take this patient's experience, for example:

> Well, one morning, I got out of bed and I realized that I was drag-
> ging my right leg. And I knew somethin' was wrong but I didn't
> know what it was. I wasn't necessarily concerned about it. So
> I got in my car and drove to Hendersonville and I told my doctor
> about that, first thing. And he asked me to walk up and down
> the corridor and outside, and he said, "Well I think you've had a
> stroke and I'm going to put you in the hospital right now." So he
> personally took me with him and signed all the papers for me.

This sense of vulnerability is indeed so strong at times that we can
experience this turning as betrayal by that which is nearer to us
than, as we might say, we are to ourselves. "My cancer came back and
I haven't been worth a damn since." "My heart just keeps acting up."
"My legs just gave way." "My hand wouldn't stop shaking." The reality
of these instances of being divided against ourselves is such a common experience, and one vested with so much power, that we have
many ways of talking about it.

We don't, however, say things like: "My head wouldn't stop feeling good." Or if someone did, it would likely be because they had a
very specific reason—a history of fiendish headaches, for example.

On the other hand, we do say things like: "My legs carried me all the way up the mountain." Or: "My hand was steady as could be." But again this will likely be in the context of a significant probability of failure, for the legs or the hands.

Reading through the transcripts one cannot but be impressed with how often the vulnerability of the body shows itself paired inextricably with the vulnerability of being a member of a family, for example, when one is planning for a family:

> My husband and I wanted to start a family and like a lot of people today, tried for a while, it didn't work out and then over time the stress begins to build. I was in a stressful job working a lot of hours and wondered to what extent the stress was contributing to the fertility problems.

And there are also times of vulnerability during the dissolution of a family:

> I started seeing her because a friend told me that what she did could help TMJ [temporomandibular joint] and I had already been to the regular dentist, to the TMJ specialist and I was still hurting and not getting a whole lot of answers.... I was in the throes of divorce and the divorce was already finalized at that point but there were still a lot of things I held in my jaw.

Our bodies also belong, in varied and specific ways, to our communities. The following is a case where the illness that motivated the patient to find his practitioner occurred at work, in fact because of his work, and then became a condition that disrupted his work life:

> I had had an incident at school where I was teaching...where I lost my temper badly. I didn't say or physically do anything but the, but the tension was, I just about exploded and from that point on I could not stop urinating. I would have to urinate over and over and over again.

7

We commonly see a clinician for disruptions in our social world that compound, or are compounded by, bodily disruptions.

And then there is violence. Violence that is never simply explained, never just damage to the physical body, but is also damage to the social-body, the mind-body, and the spirit-body:

> When I first got shot, since I couldn't get any help I got to think-ing, well you know maybe I did something that God didn't like. I mean I really went through the whole guilt.

Finally, there is the brute fact that sometimes our bodies come into contact with parts of the material world that are much more solid than we are:

> I had quite an experience about two years ago, when I was climb-ing in a remote part of Canada, Indiana Jones style, and I fell and broke the L4 in my back, and shattered my skull.

Our bodies provide access to beauty and exhilaration. But, as in this climbing example, our bodies remain vulnerable and at risk, even in the midst of beauty and exhilaration. In this particular case, exhila-ration and vulnerability led to relationships with medics and rescue personnel, neurosurgeons and hospital staff, and finally a chiroprac-tor back home. The body as one object among others, the body as social, the body wounded and healing. And it is this body that we bring to practitioners when we become patients.

VIGNETTES OF A PATIENT LIFE

One of the first things we discovered as we began interviewing was how eager people were to talk about their relationships with their clinicians. Eager, but also forthcoming; in fact, remarkably forthcom-ing. As we all know, there is a need, a longing even, to tell someone about our relationships with practitioners, about our health and our illnesses, our therapies and our recoveries. One might, in fact, consider it an essential part of healing to be able, to be allowed, and to be invited to speak in these ways.

Interviews provide a very distinctive occasion for such speaking and telling. Interviews are not narratives, strictly considered. Fundamentally, they are conversations. As such, they contain a very wide range of materials, including specific descriptions of clinician behaviors, examples and explanations of key moments, wisdom stories, anecdotes, and meta-insights. Yet most of our interviews contained multiple little stories about relationships with clinicians. We want to make our first map of patient experience by looking in some detail at the brief accounts of such episodes embedded in the interviews.[4]

We all tell stories about healthcare practitioners. If not stories about our own clinicians, then stories of someone central in our lives, central to our story—father or sister, baby or grandmother, closest friend, colleague. These stories, as we commonly relate them, tend to be small narratives, not full-blown accounts. In this section we will refer to these anecdotes as "vignettes." With this word we want to suggest in part that such stories are like scenes in a play or a movie—scenes with two or more actors in conversation with one another, in relationship with one another. We are interested here in beginning to capture the dynamic back-and-forth that goes on between clinicians and patients in healing relationships.

In our interviews, these "vignettes" are parts of longer narratives about relationships with clinicians. But in daily life, such vignettes usually stand alone—as puzzlements, as protests, as expressions of gratitude. Each, however brief or mundane, is a story of how we hold and have held our pain, and of those people who helped us hold it. Each is likewise a component of the longer story of how we deal with our stressed and often fractured world. Taken together they are components of the healing of that world.

All of us are very practiced at telling stories about doctors. Such tales are a significant genre in our culture; they circle powerful and significant territory. But in truth they mostly get in the way of fuller, deeper understandings of clinician/patient relationships. Why is that?

- They tend to run very negative. "Can you believe he did that ...?!"
- They tend to be short. The punch line comes very quickly.
- They run in clichés. "They get paid all that money and then they ..."; "He saved my life."
- They often rely on grim jokes: "What do you call a doctor who ...?"
- They prop up the tired (and unhelpful) notion of the "all-powerful doctor." That common process of canonizing or demonizing our clinicians, which denies their humanity—and ours.

And yet the impulse to tell stories about our encounters with clinicians is a terribly important one. If we follow them out, we find ourselves guided to just those places where we are most anxious or most afraid. Freud would have us recognize that it is precisely because they are so stereotypical, that such stories show us where enormous amounts of energy are stored and expended.

Unfortunately, we often "mis-tell" our doctor stories. Our stories ought to be told and listened to for clues about relationships, rather than as tales of heroes and villains (them), supplicants and victims (us). But the rules of the genre tend to keep us from going deeper, going past those familiar roles. Telling the old-fashioned doctor story, ironically enough, diverts us from a careful look at the fears and vulnerabilities that swirl around our interactions with our clinicians. We want to drive deeper and find the true sources of discomfort, to find thicker accounts of how patients and practitioners comport themselves. We think the recurring vignettes we have identified in our interviews are an excellent place to begin.

Here then are the ten types of scenes, the ten vignettes our interviewees most often shared with us. This list emerged from a detailed study of the interview transcripts.

1. Many long-term relationships with clinicians begin with a sense of "immediate recognition" on the part of the patient:
   - "I knew as soon as I met her."

- "Right when I walked into her office I felt safe."
- "When he saw my Daddy that first time, we said, 'He's the one.'"

2. Very quickly an excellent "information flow" is established:
   - "She drew those diagrams for me."
   - "He just took his time ..."
   - "After I talked with her, I knew all I needed to know."

3. Often there is "fixing" of a specific, discrete problem.
   - "And I've never had any trouble with that since."
   - "She just took that pain right out of my shoulder."
   - "You should have seen how fast my daughter recovered ..."

4. At the time when they are most vulnerable, it is of the utmost importance for the patient to feel that there's a powerful person "in my corner":
   - "He came in and said, 'Can't you find a better place for her than this?'"
   - "If they know you're Dr. H's patient ..."
   - "I don't know what I would have done without her watching out for me."

5. In explaining why they found relationships with their practitioners healing, patients described again and again the unusual "human bond" they felt with their clinician:
   - "He shared so much with me about his own illness ..."
   - "He's actually interested in me as a person!"
   - "She's a friend of our family—that's what she is."

6. Most accounts of a long-term relationship with a clinician include a heartfelt retelling of a "hard conversation":
   - "She held nothing back."
   - "He didn't pull any punches with us."
   - "They told it to us like it was."

7. Our interviewees grew especially animated when telling about the times their practitioners had gone the "extra mile":
   - "Do you know what she did?"
   - "This will show you what kind of guy he is."
   - "I couldn't believe he showed up at the ER that night."

8. Our life-story interview questions allowed our patients to share accounts of healing, accounts of "achieving wholeness," that altered their sense of what was and was not possible in their lives:
   - "Nothing has ever been the same since that conversation."
   - "I owe not just my life to her—but that of both my children."
   - "I had never dared to share the real story of my illness until ..."

9. Clinicians who could offer their "full presence" to their patients were recognized as having an unusual gift:
   - "Never met anyone like her."
   - "A poet's temperament—that's what he has ..."
   - "No matter what happens to me, he's still a great man."
   - "That's her calling—she's a healer by nature."

10. The interviews are chock-full of "wisdom stories" that offer insights into healing offered or achieved by the practitioner or the patient:
    - "Now I understand why hospice ..."
    - "She just respected my daughter's mind on this."
    - "Who else would have known to say that?"

We all recognize these vignettes. None of this is foreign to us—even if we know some only in their absence or their negation. All these vignettes touch on topics that are commonly part of the stories we tell about practitioners. But the vignettes we found in our interviews are thick with details of very particular relationships with clinicians. They arise out of specific histories and are rooted in shared experiences. Experiences that are often powerful and frequently life-changing. Here there is no repetition of stock phrases; here instead are sentences forged out of trust and commitment.

The following gives a more concrete account of these ten common vignettes by taking one interview and showing how examples of each of the vignettes can come together to tell the story of a 30-year relationship between a clinician and a patient. We will also provide, alongside each section of the interview, additional examples of each vignette drawn from other interviews.

Notice that the vignettes in the interview do not follow the order in table 1.1. Each of the ten vignettes—except for "immediate recognition"— can appear anywhere in the interview. Nevertheless, in whatever order they come, they form the building blocks of an ever-sturdier relationship. Watching them build up is one way of following the story. Another way is to say that these are the elements we should look for in every account of a long-term healing relationship with a clinician.

IMMEDIATE RECOGNITION

- *The clear sense that you're in the right place, in the first or second visit with a clinician.*

The only thing that I can remember about the [first] visit was that we were just...I was at ease. He never gave me the impression, never made me think I wanted to go look for another doctor. And he always took the time to talk to you, to learn who you were as an individual and I remember that factor, too, since I got a 30-year span, you see.

Information Flow

- *The practitioner provides a continuing stream of relevant, and requested, information.*

IMMEDIATE RECOGNITION

We walked into his room there and immediately, instantaneously, it was a total change. When he walked in...some people have a presence and attitude and he looks you right in the eye. And he had read everything. I mean there wasn't anything he didn't know about me. Then he went on to ask, "Is this your wife? How long have you been married?" Started asking some personal things, so I'm thinking to myself, I'm not quite sure what this has to do...you know, what things we were interested in, hobbies and all that stuff. It's obvious to me now that the man truly wants to know who his patients are, what drives them, what motivates them.

I have certain things that happened during that time that shows this concern and relationship. I remember I went to my gynecologist after about two years, I showed up there at my gynecologist [Dr. J] and he said, you know you've got some tumors. He said, "You know it seems like they have grown some." Dr. J was a mumbler and he'd use these big terms.

But the one thing he said, "We might wanna wait and see what happens with these tumors to see if they get larger." Well if I hadn't been in two years and I just happened to come in, I thought maybe that was an omen that I might need some medical attention. You know how you always get a second opinion? Trying to determine whether you're gonna have a hysterectomy, or whatever?

I called Dr. H for my second opinion. So I walked in and I told him why I was there and he looked at me said, "What do you want me to do?" And I said, "I want you to call Dr. J and find out what he said and tell me what he said." So Dr. H dialed him up right then, and he said, "Dr. J this is Dr. H." and so Dr. J told Dr. H all the medical terms and whatever. I remember he took out his pen and on the prescription pad, he drew a little diagram of my fallopian tubes, whatever, and explained it to me. But the one thing he says, "Are you planning on having any more children?" And I said, "Doctor, I'm out of the children business." He said, "Okay then." Because he didn't want me to have a partial hysterectomy. He said, "If you're not planning on having any more children just go ahead and have a complete hysterectomy."

In My Corner

- *The clinician is always available to serve as advocate for the patient, and at times as champion.*

So I followed his advice. But then another thing that happened with that is while I was in the

14

hospital my blood pressure went up because they took me off my medicine. They [hospital staff] said, "Your blood pressure's up a little bit." And I said, "Call Dr. H and tell him." 'Cause I'm not on it. Instead of just talking to them, I remember he came by the hospital to see me, to see how I was doing and he told 'em what medication to give me and he didn't charge for the visit.

Human Bond: I

- *There is a personal connection that goes beyond the typical clinical interactions.*

That has been one of the things that Dr. H has always been, all of these years, he was the physician for my family. After I went then I referred everybody in my family to Dr. H and it was based on the concern that he had for us as, as individual patients. I've seen him in the Kroger, he always knew me. And I was wondering as I came over here, I said he always knew me and I just wonder if he knew all his patients. Did he know everyone like he knew me and my family? I don't know whether it was a

HUMAN BOND

One time, my daughter was into drugs and she had went to Arizona on a program out there. I had to go to Dr. F, he asked me how was things going, and that day everything I had came out, I got to screaming and hollering and crying. He said, "Hold up here." He said, "Give me your hand." So I gave him my hand like that, and he said, "Why are you crying? Why are you upset like this?" And he said, "You didn't even do this when you came in and talked with me after your husband died. Now what is it?"

And I told him, I said, "He has left me and I got all of these things... and I'm the only person to make these decisions on things and take whatever's going on." And I had my daughter's two children, they was teenagers almost, and I said, "I just can't do it, I can't." [Patient laughs] He said, "Yes you can." That was one moment that a doctor, out of all of the other people talking to you... he just really put me to where I need to be. He said, "You can do it. You're a strong person. You can do it." I said, "Well, I'm not doing very well with it." He said, "Well, you're gonna be alright." And I am.

15

knack [he has] or if he just always found something he remembered each patient by.

And even on a Sunday night after the high school graduation, he was there on the campus. I said, "There goes Dr. H.," and I hollered, "Dr. H!" And he said, "Yeah I was looking for ya'll." He said, "I've already hugged Michael." That's the graduate [patient's grandson]. And Dr. H says, "I was looking for ya'll." 'Cause he was the doctor for all our family. And the last thing he told us Sunday night is, "If ya'll need me, call me."

The interview can begin with a statement of confidence—"I'm in the right place." "I've got the right people on my side." Often there is a sudden recognition that this clinician, the one before me right now, is the very one I've been hoping for. A common next turn is the sharing of information and the explanation of technical information. This is a relatively low-risk opportunity for the patient to get a sense of how this particular clinician approaches relationships with patients. Is there a sense of shared authority in the conversation? Are the explanations clear or full of jargon? Is the clinician in a big hurry or willing to take time to listen and to answer questions? All this can be ascertained in a short interaction, and can all be done while talking over medical information. These initial exchanges can be powerful, in and of themselves. But a time may come when much more intimate sharing of details of the patient's life is called for. This marks a decisive testing point for the relationship. If a human bond has been created, remarkable degrees of trust can be established at these pivotal moments.

As clinical relationships continue to develop, another turning point comes when the care for the patient is blocked in some way—by other providers, by hospital procedures, by insurance regulations, by family members. The question in the patient's mind is: "Is she going to stick up for me? I can't take on these people. This is their world, not mine. It is the doctor's world. What will she do?" When the practitioner does stand up for the patient and—most powerfully—wins the contest (for this is how it appears) for the patient, there is the sense of the patient having a champion in their corner. The relationship then takes on an added dimension of trust and gratitude. "I can count on this person. She won't leave me when I'm vulnerable."

As the trust develops and more time is spent together, there are opportunities for the practitioner and the patient to come to know more about one another. Their worlds don't just touch at clinical reference points. There's family and graduations, births and deaths, shared celebrations and shared griefs, all happening at the basic human level. Nearly all of our patients singled out this kind of bond as a particularly important aspect of a healing relationship. One might describe it as the ability to step outside the professional box—and then to be able to step right back inside. A close relationship, but professional always.

We go back now into the interview.

Extra Mile: I

- *A practitioner shows up in unexpected places, at unexpected times, going well beyond the norm.*

I: When Dr. H said, "if you need me, call me," what did that make you think or feel?

R: It just made me feel that the concern, the confidence, he's a friend. Even though he's our physician, he's our friend. After my daddy died we brought him a program of my daddy's funeral. About a year and a half later, he said to my sister, [the one who] always brought daddy to the office, "Come back to my office, I wanna show you something. Look what I still have on my desk. I have the funeral program from your dad that you brought by." He held on to it and he had it on his desk. And that just shows you the concern he has.

I: So was your dad also a patient of Dr. H's?

R: Oh yeah. You wanna hear that story?

Full Presence: I

- *The patient feels the complete attention of the clinician focused on them and their life situation.*

We were trying to find a doctor for dad that we were satisfied with, and my daddy was blind, he was a diabetic and had various health problems. So this one doctor we had would take his chart off the door and come in with his hand out looking at the chart. This particular doctor acted as though daddy couldn't hear because he was blind. He always talked to my sister, "But did he do such and such?" And she would say, "Oh Daddy, did you do so and so?" Then that doctor would write dad's prescriptions and give them to my sister. Well my sister would turn around, give it to daddy 'cause my daddy kept up with his stuff, you know he could. I said, "Daddy, I want you to see Dr. H."

Another time he called me to tell me of my breast cancer diagnosis and I made that phone call difficult by bursting out at him to hurry up and tell me what they said. Yet he approached me slowly and gently, and after a burst, he'd be silent for a moment. He knows when to be silent and let me either calm down or think or whatever. And in this case to stop my bombast. That was unappreciated at the time, but greatly appreciated later. And he continued his difficult job with care, with concern and allowing my outbursts. There wasn't much he could do about 'em. I was angry. He continued the conversation in his constantly caring voice, described the cancer slowly and helped me know I had a strong friend supporting me. Had him as a pillar, as things went along.

And I can't remember [whether] Daddy ended up with stomach cancer after he started going to Dr. H. But one of the things my sister said was that Dr. H always talked to my dad, "Reverend, how are you doing?" And when he'd write his prescriptions he'd reach over and put 'em in daddy's hands. And it was that confidence that he had. Daddy asked me, "How did you find him?" And at the end, near the end of my Daddy's life Dr. H told my, my dad, "You don't have to make an appointment. All you need to do is call the office to make sure I'm in before you come up here and then just come on, I'll work you in, I'll see you whenever you wanna come." And, you know, that's a relationship that most times you can't get.

Hard Conversations: I

- *The practitioner is right there to help the patient handle bad news and make tough choices.*

R: And then we went through end-of-life transitions when my mother died and then also my little sister died. We went through that with Dr. H. He sat down and explained it all to us.

I: Anything else that he did that you found especially helpful during those end-of-life transitions?

Extra Mile: II

R: When my mother had a stroke at my daughter's house on a Saturday because I and another sister had gone to a basketball game. While we were there they paged us. This was before cell phones. So when the EMTs arrived she said, "I want to go to St. Luke's because that's where Dr. H is." This is like 11:00 at night, on a Saturday. The EMT said, "We can take her to Central. That's the closest place." She says, "No,

HARD CONVERSATION

So Dr. Smith had his secretary call me: "Come downtown tomorrow." And I knew it wasn't anything good going to come out of it. And he said, "Jim, I've been your doctor and I sincerely like you." He said, "But what you did, you could have killed yourself. And I don't want to stay around and watch you die. If you're going to continue to drink, just go out there and tell 'em to take you off my patient list because I don't want to see it." And damn, that sounded serious as hell to me. You know, the guy's been my doctor for years, put that kind of stuff on me. That's shootin' pretty damn straight in the belly. Since that day I've been off the booze.

I want to go to St. Luke's, that's where Dr. H is." The EMT said, "Well lady, let me tell you, he will not come out. You know he's not gonna come out tonight to the hospital." She says, "That's where I wanna go." So they said "Fine," and took my mother to St. Luke's. And even before the EMTs could leave, Dr. H was there.

Hard Conversations: II

R: And then during the time after mother had the strokes Dr. H called us all in. And he made sure everybody was there, including the sister who helped with my mother and another sister who likes to not be around things like this. Dr. H said, "I want Bessie [the second sister] there. So you tell her she's got to come. We're gonna have a discussion." Because he knew Bessie wouldn't show up 'cause she's a little skittish. So when we had that consultation about taking the tubes out and everything, Dr. H didn't know what was gonna happen. But then momma just raised up and started talking after that. Then momma had more mini-strokes and Dr. H recommended Graceland for rehab. And then at the end he recommended Clearwater Hospice. And at that time I had had some experience with hospice, I knew a little about it, but we didn't know a whole lot about it. But because he recommended hospice care, we said okay. And it was a good experience.

Typically the relationship is already on solid footing when the clinician does something truly exceptional, at an unusual time or place. Not just an exceptional job with a procedure or an office visit. When we speak of going the extra mile, we tell stories about our practitioners showing up in the emergency room late at night or on a weekend. We're thinking of a reassuring phone call that comes while the clinician is on vacation. We think of the doctor who stays at the hospital far longer than expected or even necessary. At these times a whole new shared sense of the meaning of their relationship is revealed to the clinician and patient.

A relationship can expand only to the range of presence each person brings to it. With the phrase "full presence" we are trying to indicate a person willing and able to listen with their whole being. Not just with the eyes and ears of a clinician, but with a full-body focus on the patient. Invited in this way, we as patients can often find the trust and courage to step up and be present. It is hard, given the power differentials, for the patient to call forth "full presence" from a clinician. But certainly the patient can be prepared to respond and can try to be fully present to herself. For this is not just something one person offers another, it is something one offers oneself as well. Here, in moments of "full presence," lies the possibility for the patient-practitioner relationship to move to levels of recognition that would be unusual in any human relationship.

As patient and practitioner continue to work together, experiences of the kind we describe in our vignettes tend to recur. So in our interview we find now a second instance of the patient feeling that her doctor is "in her corner." It is this very repetition of the positive, powerful experience that demonstrates to the patient the fundamental reliability of her clinician, which in turn allows still more trust to develop.

And then inevitably comes one of the tragic events that cut across a life: the disabling accident, the discovery of a terminal disease, the confirmation of a diagnosis of a debilitating chronic or progressive illness. The often wrenching process of accompanying the dying. The death—whether sudden or long-expected—of a parent, a spouse, a child. These are a part of every long-term relationship between a patient and a healthcare provider. And in such times, how much can be spoken? And in what way? How much honesty and detail and depth can conversations between a patient and a practitioner hold? The handling of what we call "hard conversations" was a key test of their relationships with clinicians for nearly every one of our patients. And what counts as doing it well? Honesty. Pulling no punches. Clarity. Compassion and kindness. A sense of shared loss, shared grief. "We're human being in this together, and it hurts." And then, perhaps most important of all, not being abandoned. "Yes this is awful, but I will stay here with you." This is what we all want to hear.

And then, again, the "extra mile." And then again, more "hard conversations," and over the years the relationship becomes richer and more rewarding.

We go once more back into our interview.

Full Presence: II

Now I understand fully what hospice is all about. When my little sister got to the end of life, Dr. H told us on a Friday, "Just call all her friends and tell them tell 'em if they want to see her to come on over the weekend. And I want to talk with you all on Monday at 1:00." And so we all gathered at 1:00 on that Monday and he says, "You know Maggie is at the end and we wanna take her off life support." And one of my sisters says, "Well doctor, this is my granddaughter's birthday. If there's anyway possible, we do not want Maggie to die on that child's birthday." And he didn't say nothing really. He just kinda nodded. And then so they did not take her off life support until the next day, after my granddaughter's birthday. You know, he honored that request.

Achieving Wholeness

- *Stories about the clinician's role in major turning points in the course of a patient's illness.*

We feel like Dr. H was very honest with us and he had a concern with us. We liked the fact that he was up front with us when he called us in. He sat down and he was very honest with the diagnosis and what was gonna happen. And we laughed, we'd talk about the healthcare bill and the end of life, and Sarah Palin says the "death panels," and we said, "Yeah, if you wanna call it that, but everybody's gonna have one."

Somebody has to sit down and there are decisions to be made you know and, and it's good for somebody to sit there and talk to you about it. But those are special moments because he sat there and he explained everything to us, what was happening and that we'd done all we can do and we'd sat there and looked at, especially my little sister, at the monitor you know and, and I knew she was just with us only, just by the life-supports. But he made the transition very painless—well, not painless, but it was easier to understand.

Human Bond: II

I: You've already talked about some other physicians or clinicians that you've had relationships with.

R: I guess I always thought that the physicians didn't become attached nowadays. Is Dr. H attached to our family? I don't know. We think he is and that's the only thing that's important. I guess we just grew up with him, you know? And I would hear him in the other room, not the conversation verbatim, but I could hear the little laughter, the making the patients feel at ease and I think that's more the healing process.

I: You've heard him with other patients in other exam rooms?

R: Yeah and the laughter, that's the way I feel about [his] showing concern.

ACHIEVING WHOLENESS

When he started talking about "How's your exercise? How do you eat?" About your need for a counselor. You began to think, "Well he's not just dealing with my pain. He's seeing me as a whole person." And I thought, "I am a whole person. I can be a whole person again." I don't wanna be remembered as the woman on the corner that got shot in the head. I really wanna be remembered as more than that 'cause I've always been more than that.

That was probably my first day of saying, "Thank you, Jesus. Thank you for the whole person." Like an old mule...I think I just took my blinders off and thought, "Wow, there can be more to this than just getting shot."

Fixing

FIXING

- *A successful, specific treatment of a specific, isolated problem.*

He said to me, "Okay, this is the deal." He did this ultrasound or whatever it is. He said, "I know exactly what the problem is here." He put a catheter in and drained an enormous amount of fluid from me.

I: Are there any other important moments or events with Dr. H that you feel capture the relationship?

R: I remember this one. My daughter was getting married and she got home Tuesday before the wedding. She had this cold and was just stopped up and everything, so she went to Dr. H. Now she lived out of town, I called him and he said, "Yep, tell her to come on." And he looked at her and she said, "Doctor I'm getting married on Friday night and I want you to get me well." And he laughed, but that was the kind of relationship that we had. Anyway, whatever he gave her, she was well by Friday. Maybe just her confidence that she would get better. He might have just gave her one of those, what kind of pills you call 'em?

I: Placebo?

R: Yeah, he might have given her one of them. [Patient laughs] That's not important what kind of pill it was, it was a pill.

Wisdom Story

- *Insights into healing offered or achieved by the practitioner or the patient.*

As I look back over it, the 30 years, the confidence—I think that's 90 to 95 percent of the healing process. It goes back to being raised in the country and whatever my grandmother would give me, I always felt like she could make me well. It's this kind of confidence...'cause you just say, whatever he thinks or whatever he says, for lack of a better term, is law and gospel. It's the confidence level. I found a doctor and I think that's what, what you really need, a doctor that you have confidence in.

When patients and clinicians have gone through a lot together, they are often both blessed with moments of insight, moments when something either the clinician or the patient says or does offers a glimpse into life's core mysteries. When our interviewees were giving accounts of such moments, we knew we were being entrusted with "wisdom stories." These stories were often about wisdom shown by the clinician in a particular encounter, and just as often about a realization the patient comes to later.

Many of the most moving passages in our interviews are those in which patients talk about pivotal healing events,

WISDOM STORY

They came up and told me they found this cancer and, and apparently in the lobe down here. But then, up here, there's a mass that they're concerned with because it could push sidewards against the windpipe. I will be 89 in about two weeks, and so, I said, "You all just forget it 'cause that's what I'm gonna do." I've seen the surgery; I've seen the chemo and the radiation. I have absolutely no responsibilities. I don't have anybody I have to take care of, or anybody depending on me. And at my age, 88 then, I said, "Just forget it. We'll go out with this. It's been fun. It's been great. But I would far rather go." I said, "I never have been afraid of death."

activities, or experiences. At some point along the way the patient undergoes a shift in their sense of life that is about more than just being fixed or cured. Unexpected openings and unexpected healers appear. One's sense of what is possible in life is transformed. What had been lived as a wound is reconceived as a breaking-through, a gift, or even a blessing. A new wholeness is achieved. These shifts, these pivotal movements, are always the fruit of exceptional trust and understanding and shared confidence between patient and practitioner.

One thing we all expect our healthcare providers to do is to fix things. Most of our interviews included accounts of clinicians doing very specific things, in answer to specific time-bound crises: maybe

a procedure; maybe a prescription. Typically, however, our interviewees didn't spend a lot of time talking about the "fixing" their practitioners did. In part, this had to do with the nature of the questions
we asked—and of those we didn't. But studying the transcripts of
the interviews, we got the clear impression that fixing was expected.
It was the restoring to wholeness that was special.

This makes fundamental sense. The assumption tends to be: "Of
course they can fix it; that's what they trained to do." The idea being
that any competent clinician ought to be able to do "x" and "y," even
when "x" might be a heart transplant. But when it comes to healing
and to wisdom, "Now that's quite a different thing."

This book, then, seeks to answer a fundamental but largely unexplored question: What do patients see as the core elements in forming healing relationships with their healthcare providers? And this
leads to a set of correlative questions: What practitioner traits are
conducive to establishing healing relationships and what are the barriers to such relationships? How do clinician-patient interactions figure into the larger life of patients outside the clinical setting? With
these questions in mind, and the foundational work we have done
in this chapter, we are now ready to begin a systematic and detailed
examination of what our interviewees have to teach us.

[2]

CLINICAL SPACE AND
TRAITS OF HEALING

In this chapter we examine how clinicians create therapeutic alliances. First we will discuss the capacity practitioners have to "make a space" for healing to happen. This will lead into a discussion of particular clinician skills and traits that our patient informants said were most important to them. We will begin by naming and describing the larger clinician capacity that allows these traits to function therapeutically. Our interest is not simply in the fact that successful practitioners are found to be trustworthy, attentive, and caring. The decisive feature here is that the actions and attitudes that manifest in such clinician traits occur in what for most of us remain unusual circumstances. Skilled clinicians establish a highly specialized physical and psychological space into which they receive their patients and attend to their vulnerabilities. Patients also have a role in sustaining this interpersonal healing sphere, but the initial, decisive work is done by the clinician. Our phrase for this capacity is "holding clinical space."[1] It is an active, intentional, and enabling capacity that allows for everything else of importance in health care to happen.

We often speak of people who can "hold a room," meaning they are engaging, magnetic people who are able to sustain the focus and attention of others to an exceptional degree. This phrase is often used to describe political or other public figures, but it is also used in social, religious, and a variety of other contexts. Skilled clinicians have similar powers, but the setting and purpose of their work means that they can hold a space that is conducive to therapy, to a healing experience for their patients.

The metaphor of holding clinical space is rooted in the clinician's ability to protect, support, and attend to those who need care. This holding ability is perhaps the most basic element, actually a precondition, for healing in health care. The intimacy suggested by *holding* reinforces that clinical space is, ideally, a place for receiving us when we are at our most vulnerable. We all know what this means, for we quite regularly hold, and hold on, to one other, both literally and figuratively.[2] We hold babies to our chest; we hold hands as we walk; we hold ideas, fears, and hopes with and for our loved ones. Sometimes with great care, other times carelessly. The intimacy suggested by *holding* is appropriate here, aptly pointing to the fragility of persons who seek the shelter of clinical space and the advocacy it affords. Clinicians hold our arms and legs as well as our fears of illness and hopes for cure.

DEVELOPING BODILY RAPPORT

Creating clinical space begins with the placement and then the movement of the bodies of the people involved. If holding clinical space is the basic precondition for healing, developing bodily rapport is the first expression of professional responsiveness. Bodily rapport is the careful coordination of bodies in time and space for the purpose of healing. From the moment the patient enters an examination room, even before the clinician arrives, they are listening and looking and reading *everything* around them, always with the fundamental question: Will this be a person or a place responsive to my needs? Once the clinician arrives, patients are often aware that the clock is ticking and they notice how their practitioner handles clinical time. Clinicians who are skilled at developing bodily rapport prepare and plan the movements—beginnings, endings, and the critical steps in between—of the visit.

Our interviewees were keenly aware that clinicians must distribute their time across multiple patients. They appreciated practitioners who guided them through a clinic visit, carefully moving the interaction from beginning to end. Patients noted—sometimes in great detail—how a visit began and the words or gestures that a practitioner used to mark the beginning of their interaction. This patient, who had a routine clinic visit the same day as our interview, gives a number of details about what the clinician says and does at the beginning of the visit to send the message that they won't be rushed. The cumulative effect is that the patient feels "calm," which echoes the calmness of the clinician.

> R: But I would say that the, the interesting thing about Dr. James is he never seems to be in any rush, so you're calm, you feel calm to start with, there's no pressure on you.
> I: Okay, if you were to paint the picture of what it's like …
> R: He starts, he looks over the vital signs that they've already taken, the nurse has already gotten everything together that he needs, the basic data and then he says, if I'm in there just for a checkup like this morning, he says, "Okay everything looks pretty good, but let's check a few things," and he'll walk across the room, he's slowly just kinda having me do things.

The pace at which this physician begins and moves through the physical exam sends the message that they are not going to rush through the visit.

> He says, "How about that? How's that feeling?" I said fine. He said, "What's wrong? Got any problems?" I said, "Well, a little bit in my back, but nothing serious." So he had me do some turns and things. He said, "Well, if it gets any worse, we may have to think about it a little more, but it's not enough to worry. Does it bother you at the end of the day?" And I said, "No." He says, "Good, let's leave it alone for now." He doesn't rush into things.

The relationship between time and the deeper patient-clinician relationship is not simple. Time has quantitative and qualitative dimensions. Slower is not always better. The skill of beginning and moving through a clinic visit does not have a definitive formula. It does require the awareness of how words and movements affect patients' perception of pace. Sometimes the length of the clinical interaction is a critical element. But far more often the sense of having "plenty of time" has to do with the way clinicians establish a human rhythm for the visit. Bodily time is not the same as clock time. Extraordinary clinicians are ones who can keep track of both kinds, while holding fast to the priority of the time we carry in our bodies.

And then there is space: the moment the clinician enters the room, many things begin to happen, instantaneously and simultaneously. The way the bodies of the clinician and the patient are initially arranged, even before the talking begins, is itself a communication of major importance, one that provides an interpretive field for everything that comes after. How bodies are positioned and where they are located are key components in any interaction, but these dynamics are of primary importance in healthcare settings. Patients of course care a great deal about what is done to their bodies and are understandably quite mindful of what the clinician is doing with his or her body. They note whether a clinician is sitting or standing, moving or still, looking or not looking at them, keeping or closing distance. These bodily communications send messages about a wide range of factors, including warmth or coolness, trust or wariness, interest or lack of interest in being there. Skilled practitioners can quickly establish a physical alignment with patients and turn it toward the larger goal of health.

"Come in, sit down, and look me in the eye." Dozens of patients gave us almost this exact formula. Why does this familiar injunction come up time and time again when talking with patients about their practitioners? We would suggest that it is in part due to the role of eye contact, sitting down, and an appropriate handshake or touch on the shoulder for establishing the bodily rapport between practitioner and patient that must be developed for clinical space to be physically and emotionally safe.

Simple and routine behaviors play a decisive role in creating a safe clinical space. Guiding the patient in making the transition from ordinary, daily routines into the often anxiety-provoking and uncomfortably intimate encounters is a critical skill for practitioners. Holding clinical space begins with the familiar and continues with steady, uncomplicated presence. As patients enter and share this space with their clinicians they become emotionally and physically prepared for the kinds of questions and touching that will likely occur as an appointment progresses.[3]

Skillful practitioners communicate with their bodies that their attention is focused on this patient, in this room, at this time. One patient stated that without eye contact, "you're not really with me." Several patients reported that steady eye contact was a sign of the clinician's confidence and competence. And, as one might expect, studies have shown that sitting down serves as a gateway action that supports many other beneficial clinical behaviors.[4] As one medical resident put it, "I've noticed that whenever I sit down I listen more."[5]

Even more essential for establishing bodily rapport is appropriate touching. The power of touch both to cause and to relieve pain makes it a complicated action for both parties. Intentions and trust matter a great deal.

I: So it's important to touch patients in ways that are healing, with permission.

R: Yeah and I think it's a difficult thing because there's also this sense of ethical boundaries in terms of touch.... But on the other hand it's meant a lot to me if I was in the hospital and one of my doctors come and just takes my hand, just as a sign of support rather than, "Let me check your fingernails to check your oxygen level." It says, "I care about you as a person" rather than "I really need to check something about the biology here."

I: But you also recognize the need for the boundary and that the clinician needs to be able to navigate that space.

R: Yeah and I really respect clinicians who can navigate that line between them because I know it is difficult, but certainly most

of my growing up experience is clinicians would err on the
side of the complete lack of compassion or lack of any kind of
touch or contact that would be reassuring or calming.

Clinical touch can be part of an examination. It can also serve
to break the isolation patients so often feel when they are in the
throes of illness and treatment. One hospice patient put it this way:
"Dr. Bergson walked in the office, and gave me a big hug. It's been a
long time since I've been hugged."

Closing the distance to touch a patient must be done with intention, skill, and great care. Yet painful touch is often necessary for
healing. Skilled practitioners know that even that kind of touching
can be done with compassion:

> This one therapist told me to do what I could do, and he'd would
> take me as far as I could go. He could tell the therapy was very
> painful. He nearly had tears in his eyes, he said, "I really hate to
> hurt you." You know that made me feel good, but I wanted to be
> hurt if it was gonna do any good. He showed sympathy. I just
> could tell from his attitude that he really wanted to help.

And then there are those times that just closing the distance
between patient and provider can have the effect of a warm embrace.
The following patient had a complicated medical history, a large sampling of providers, and a penchant for analyzing physician behavior.
Her praise for providers was often parsimonious. But not in this case.

> Just—his smile, eyes, level voice, it fluctuates a little, but it's
> always kind and I highlighted that because [his voice] is so big.
> He has shown appropriate concern when something new occurs,
> I can see it on his face, I can see it in his body language, he'll look
> concerned and lean slightly toward me. It's almost a hug.

Receiving patient vulnerability requires respectful and confident
bodily comportment of clinicians. If vulnerability and responsiveness

are the core structure of healthcare ethics—as we are proposing—then *bodily rapport is the most basic element of professional responsiveness*.

PARTICULAR CLINICIAN TRAITS THAT HEAL

We now turn from the overall importance of the clinician's ability to hold a clinical space for healing to a consideration of particular actions and attitudes that are prominent both in establishing clinical space and in nurturing healing relationships within that space. We consistently asked our patient interviewees what it is that clinicians say and do that promotes healing relationships. Sometimes they responded with reports of specific words and actions, in scenes and vignettes such as the ones we discussed in chapter 1. But just as often they spoke in generic, summary terms about qualities of heart and mind that they attributed to their clinicians. In our discussion below we use the word "trait" as a shorthand reference to these practitioner qualities and characteristics, mindful that they are always traceable to specific incidents in patients' stories.

Our focus is on the most frequently mentioned traits. We also take up several of the traits in groups of twos and threes for analysis. We do this to emphasize that the traits are not isolated characteristics, but are always embodied in some larger activity. The patients named these particular traits precisely because they had seen them in action. The traits are listed in Table 2.1 in the order of their frequency—ranked, that is, by the number of patients who noted each one as important.

Calmness

A very wise person we interviewed explained how for her the clinician's body language and overall demeanor work as a critical element in healing. Some clinicians, she said, have too much nervous energy.

> They're always fussing with things on their desk, or tapping their feet, or rearranging papers, or looking around. If they could just be still and focused it creates an envelope in which it's okay to be

Table 2.1 POSITIVE CLINICIAN TRAITS

Clinician Traits	Frequency
Caring, empathy, compassion	43
Attentive or broader awareness	33
Accessibility	28
Advocacy	25
Honesty	25
Trustworthy, good judgment	25
Calm, puts patient at ease	24
Respectful	20
Openness	20
Warmth	18
Confidence	17
Humorous	16
Shared authority	13
Humility	12
Spiritual, religious	8
Cheerful or positive demeanor	7
Technical competence	6

there... [and when that envelope is created] it has encouraged me to be completely honest about what's going on.

Both ancient and contemporary clinicians commend the kind of interior serenity this patient points to. In "On the Physician," Hippocrates advises that physicians always be well kempt, honest, *calm*, understanding, and serious (emphasis added).[6] Among contemporary physician writers, Jerome Groopman commends calmness as a factor in helping to avoid errors in judgment.[7] Beyond these cognitive advantages for a clinician, of interest here is how stillness and tranquility can elicit confidence in patients and enable a more thorough history and a more collaborative engagement. Emotions are contagious, and calmness in the clinician can translate into a similar state for patients and their families. Going back to our earlier analysis, we could say that calmness enhances bodily rapport, while creating a safe space to hold the anxieties, fears, and concerns of patients in a way that leads to healing.

Attentiveness and Broader Awareness

I think that a clinician of any kind somehow has to clear his or her head, and what's in front of them, what's in the room, is all that matters.

More than half the interviewees spoke of a trait in their providers that we came to understand as attentiveness. These clinicians demonstrated a broad range of awareness, ranging far beyond knowledge of the pathophysiology of a given disease. At times this was most evident in a practitioner's ability to focus in, to block out everything but the patient being seen right then. At other times, this was expressed in the clinician's willingness to follow through with courses of therapy, attending to the patient's needs over the course of long illness episodes. At still other times, it was taking special care with a family member or another primary caregiver.

One patient recalls observing when his doctor was taking the initial history.

And I was watching the whole time he was asking questions and he would tell you why he was asking the questions. He wouldn't tell you [all the time], but I could just tell by his demeanor that this was a man who was interested.

Seeking further descriptions, we asked: "How does this attentiveness show itself?" One common indicator was the thoroughness with which the patient's questions were answered: "[She] answered every question that my wife and I could possibly have, very patiently, in words or terms we could explain." Another factor was the appreciation of nonmedical influences on the course of a therapy. What follows is the testimony of a hospice patient. Her patient's daughter is the first speaker.

R2: And then they're [also] concerned about me, making sure that my health is—that I can be able to take care of her [the patient], that I'm not overloaded.

I: So they're seeing the family picture. [Addressing the patient] They aren't just focused on you, but are trying to get the whole picture.

R: And then they contact my children. They want them to be involved, and be up to date with what's going on.

Sometimes attentiveness is very simply a willingness to suspend a technical task to just be with a patient.

He is so tuned in to what you're going through. You know I had cancer and he had to refer me to a specialist, and he was right there in surgery with me. And the doctor who did the surgery goes, "I don't understand the connection between you." I said, "And you never will."

The patient's response shows how prized her relationship with her primary provider is.

Honesty and Trust

I don't know how I could have a relationship with somebody in the medical profession that I didn't trust, or didn't feel that when they walk in this front door, I'm their main concern.

Honesty and its synonyms, such as candor, were mentioned by 25 of our 58 informants. Trust was also mentioned a similar number of times, often by the same patients.

I: If you were in a room of medical and nursing students, and you were trying to teach them something about building a good relationship with their patients, what would you tell them?

R: I would tell them to come straight, they need to come straight to people, don't be in there beating around the bush.

Honesty or candor at the beginning of a relationship invites and builds trust, and trust then leads to a deeper candor on the part of the patient regarding their larger concerns. To begin simply, patients often realize that the truth, even when it is bad news, is better than catastrophic imaginings. One cancer patient put it this way: "I would rather know and have the truth than to sit at home and worry and conjure up things." Our patient informants were certainly not suggesting their clinicians do what has been colorfully described as "truth-dumping." While insisting that truthfulness is a basic condition of relationships with clinicians, they were also clear that they preferred that the necessary truth always be relayed with courtesy, tact, and whatever hope could be reasonably entertained.

People need to have some understanding of what's wrong with them. What can and can't be done, I mean maybe this is a lot to ask of a doctor, but I don't think it is. I think it's part of their job.

One fear is that the clinician will conceal bad news with jargon, or words that obfuscate rather than reveal.

I think sometimes people hide, not just doctors; lawyers do this too and politicians do it all the time...hide beyond words that confuse people. You know, you sort of stay back. That's what I like about Dr. Burns. He's very open. And he tells you what he wants you to know, and what you need to know. You got some question and he'll say, "Yes, we can work on that."

One of the noticeable things in many patient narratives is the way truth and candor can reduce the distance between clinician and patient and form a common bond for whatever comes next.

R: He is letting you know that he is aware of your situation and if you will just work with him, there are things we can do. And he told me up front that this will be a lifelong thing. It won't get well, but he can make it better.

I: And you appreciated that honesty?

R: I did. Because if you are looking to get well immediately and it's not going to happen that would be as devastating as not knowing what was going on.

It is obviously counterproductive for patients both when they do not know what their prognosis is, and when they entertain false hopes for a quick fix.

Noteworthy as well were conversations in which clinicians were candid about their own limitations. Here is one example, told by a patient whose diagnosis was elusive to her primary care practitioner. The patient and her daughter are talking about their response to his acknowledgment of his own limitations.

R: He did all the things he could think of and were available, and he said, "I'm going to send you to somebody that knows more than I do." I don't think he had any frustration, God love him.

R2: I think he felt bad about it…that he couldn't make the diagnosis.

R: He told me, "I just can't find it; it's time that we sent you to somebody else. I can't tell you what you've got. It's time to go further."

R2: And he has to this day kept up with her case even though he does not treat her at all.

The idea that truth and candor build relationships was never better expressed in our interviews than by those facing a terminal illness. There was, for example, a hospice patient with inoperable lung cancer whose message to us was that truth on the part of the clinician invites reciprocity from the patient. "They level with me, and that's what I ask. When the hospice doctor came, I said, 'I want you to look me in the eye, I want you to be blunt and to the point (laughs), and I will do the same for you.'"

Accessibility and Advocacy

It's very easy to get lost in the system.

More than half our patients told stories about their access to clinicians, often in tones of surprise and always with appreciation. Cell phones and e-mails were mentioned frequently, as well as the clinician's receptivity to being called on off-days or inconvenient hours. Here a patient tells of being in the UK and calling her clinician after discovering a lump in her breast.

> When I was concerned I might have breast cancer, I had a mammogram five months before, and nothing was there. And I always went to the same diagnostic clinic...and I found the tumor myself, I was in England and I picked up the phone in England and called him at his office, [then] I called him at home cause it was that time [time difference of six hours]. He was just so concerned, wanting to know when I would be back. I don't know if he had to change his schedule or not, but when I walked in [upon her return] he saw me immediately.... They skipped the mammogram, sent me for a sonogram...and had me in the surgeon's office the next morning.

Another patient told in a matter of fact way that she has called her clinician several times at night. Her narrative indicates the warmth and closeness that allow this degree of accessibility.

> R: The first impression, the way he came in here, the way he talked to me, I just fell in love with him. I fell completely in love with him as a physician. His bedside manner was one of the best.
> I: What is it that he does?
> R: I can talk to Dr. Rick about anything. I have called Dr. Rick at 2:00 and 3:00 in the morning on his home phone.

And this patient continued her narration to be sure the interviewer understood that access was not contingent on her ability to pay for her care. Here access translated into advocacy and patient loyalty. "My insurance ran out when my husband left his job, but Dr. Rick has never turned his back on me, not one time."

Patients are also sensitive about how questions of access are approached by their clinicians. This patient parses carefully the terms offered to her.

There's a lot of confusion over the words "want" and "need," and if a doctor says, "Call me if you need me," I will sit at home saying, "Well I really don't need him." And if the doctor says, "Call me if you want," I sit at home thinking, I don't know what "want" is, I don't know what "need" is, and it is confusing. And I think patients might call too often with the "want" word, and too little with the "need" word. So I suggest the clinician say something like, "Call me if you have a question, okay?" And the "okay" is, "I really mean it."

Access also has psychological dimensions. One patient said she always felt that her practitioner held a "nonjudgmental" space for her to return to. For other patients it was their clinicians' willingness to adjust schedules for them: "I'll work you in." An older patient who transferred to a new practitioner upon the closing of a practice spoke of being surprised and happy that her retired clinician called to inquire about how she was doing. One patient talked about her sadness that her clinician was retiring but noted that he said at their last meeting, "If you need me, call me." Still others talked about receiving unsolicited phone calls from their clinician, often to follow up after an office visit.

Some of the stories we were told could be categorized in so many domains of analysis that it becomes hard to single out one theme or one provider trait over another. One such story came from a patient who had experienced major traumas, both physical and psychological. Self-sufficient, largely through her own wits and persistence, she had been shot in the face by a member of her family. She had been handled in a less than respectful way when initially treated in the emergency department. Afterward, she routinely received indifferent care. And, on top of that, she was consistently stigmatized as she sought assistance. She finally reached a clinician who truly received her.

> Yeah, that had never been spoken of, because of my shame, and that's when I opened up. The first time I met with Dr. Frazer, I had prayed, "Will you get me to a doctor who will help me, I will start from scratch and tell him everything." I had never bothered to tell anybody because I was so ashamed, and I will never forget sitting in that office, and that man has the kindest eyes I had ever looked into, and when he offered me a tissue, and I said, I'm so sorry because it's hard to tell people what you've lived through, and things you don't want people to know. And I'll never forget him saying, "There is nobody here gonna hurt you, we're going to help you, and you'll be loved here." I never had a doctor say that in my whole life. I understand that to be a doctor you have to go to school a long time, but Dr. Frazer has a heart, and that's what doctors should have.... He's kind and he's gentle and he looks at the person, he don't just look at what the folder says, and that makes the difference.

Because of the enormous care he demonstrated, and because of his willingness to advocate for her, this clinician sparked a new level of trust in this patient and enabled her return to a full life.

Caring, Empathy, Compassion

You think from the first time he talks to you that he cares.
Let them see you have a heart. [a patient's advice to young clinicians]

We have categorized under this heading many stories that relate generally to caring, showing deep concern, exercising empathy, and practicing compassion. This is a set of terms that can mean many different things. Unsurprising yet noteworthy is the fact that this cluster of traits was at the top of the list of provider qualities that enable or activate a healing response. We will disaggregate them, and then define them more closely as we proceed in this section.

Caring

Here a hospice patient speaks about the nurse who visited her at home:

> I: So, what makes her good? What does she do that makes her good?
>
> R: She cares.

And how is care communicated? Sometimes it comes across in how the clinician touches the patient, in both a physical and an emotional sense. Here an elderly patient, with his wife present for the interview, describes how he is treated by his family physician.

> R: When I first met Dr. Lyons, he examined me, and after the exam we talked. I realized he had the heart of some of our doctors back home [this couple had spent most of their lives abroad]. And that's what drew me to him.
>
> R2: That's a good word; I felt that he cared.
>
> R: I think all doctors want to help their patients.... Dr. Lyons goes beyond that; he wants to help the person other than just medically.
>
> I: And you know that because of the way he talks to you, and also the ways he touches you when he's examining you?
>
> R2: He's just very kind.

"Having a heart" is a continuing thread and an *Ur*-theme for many of the narratives we heard. At the close of many interviews we asked each of our patient informants what advice they would offer to medical students and other clinicians in training. What should we tell students to do to facilitate and enhance therapeutic interactions with their patients? One patient's answer was typical of the advice many others gave: "I would tell them, listen, first thing you can do is let them know you have a heart, let them see your heart. And you do that by showing compassion." She goes on to develop this theme in some detail.

> Show 'em, "I'm here to help you, and I want to be more than just your doctor." So when the doctor comes in, and asks, "What's going on?"...90% [of patients] won't tell their doctors what is really going on, because he doesn't really want to know. [Show the patient] that you really want to know, that it's not just one of the questions on the questionnaire.... they'll give you penicillin, and then you feel bad, or you're not taking it, or you're depressed, and you're not going to get well. So I think the one thing is just let 'em know you care, and they'll tell you, once they know you really care.

Those familiar with the history of medical ethics will recognize in the quote above a twenty-first-century patient's version of the famous maxim of Dr. Francis Peabody, found in a 1927 address he gave to his students at Boston City Hospital: "The secret of the care of the patient is in caring for the patient."[8] This quote has been cited so often it has become a cliché. But seldom quoted are the insights that provided the context of Peabody's memorable aphorism.

> In all your patients whose symptoms are of functional origin, the whole problem of diagnosis and treatment depends on your insight into the patient's character and personal life, and in every case of organic disease there are complex interactions between the pathologic processes and the intellectual processes which you must appreciate and consider if you are to be a wise clinician.

Time, sympathy, understanding, and "interest in humanity" comprise the list of traits Peabody recommended to the novice clinicians in his charge. He urged appreciation for the intrinsic rewards of practicing these traits, speaking of "that personal bond which forms the greatest satisfaction of the practice of medicine." And going further, he underscored the contribution of these four traits to higher-quality care, asserting that physicians who attempt to practice while neglecting these are "unscientific."[9] Early twenty-first-century technologies of neuroimaging, which allow us to picture the physiological registers of emotional resonance between humans, provide recent testimony to the truth of what Peabody said in 1927—and in so doing confirm what our patient informants told us in 2010.

Empathy

Here a cardiac patient is describing his physician. He has a friend present for the interview.

> R: Well, some people have empathy.
> R2: Very strong empathy with other people.
> R: Dr. Thomson [the patient's cardiologist] is like that. That's as much as I can explain. He's just a delightful man; it's a pleasure to be his patient really. He empathizes, and he's cheerful, and lighthearted, and he's a likable man.

Searching for the right word in a field of adjectives to designate the obvious warmth of this relationship, the patient returns to empathy as a dominant theme. Empathy is a much misunderstood capacity, yet clearly one that is decisive in healing relationships of all kinds. Taking a moment, then, to recover a more precise sense of the term and delineate the differences between empathy and its near cousins will be a useful undertaking.

One of the most insightful analyses of empathy comes from physician Richard Sobel in a 2008 article in *Perspectives in Biology and Medicine*. Empathy, Sobel claims, is "the ability of an individual to discern, both cognitively and emotionally, what another person is thinking or feeling at a particular moment in time."[10] Empathy always involves some distance between people. It is not a merging of feelings, nor is its force exclusively, or even primarily, emotional.

Sympathy, Sobel says, is identity of feeling—feeling what the other person feels, as in the hackneyed phrase, "I feel your pain"; but it is also captured in the more customary and everyday experience of laughing or crying spontaneously when others do so. Feelings often have this mirroring valence, such that we naturally tend to be sad when others are, and happy when the social context is a joyous one. This contagiousness, what might be described as "affective echoing," is an everyday experience. Empathy, by contrast, is reserved for a more imaginative movement, in which identity of feeling is not paramount—a movement marked instead by the recognition of the situation of the other person. When empathy is exercised, according to Sobel, the other person is perceived as just as alive and vital as oneself, but as clearly distinct from oneself.[11]

It is clear from our interviews that the sort of trait our informants want to signal through the term "empathy" was just this capacity on the part of their clinicians to understand them as people, to get a glimpse of their lives from the inside—something far more than a clinician who simply mirrors their feelings. Empathy, our participants told us, allowed them to feel like they were known to their clinician, and known in a way similar to the way they know themselves. Another way to mark the difference between empathy and sympathy is through how these two capacities are expressed. A patient may know that a clinician sympathizes with them, for example, if they tear up when the patient cries, or cries with the family when lifesaving therapy fails. And without question, this is valued. The expression of empathy, by contrast, is primarily the capacity for a careful attentiveness, and it shows in the effort it takes to make an imaginative leap into the patient's situation, to see life from her perspective, to walk in her shoes. Empathy is a more specific, more self-conscious, and more arduous skill to employ.[12]

Psychotherapist Piero Ferrucci observes that studies have shown that "the more empathic a doctor is, the more her patients see her as competent."[13] We would add to this observation: the more empathic a doctor is the more likely she is to *be* competent, where competence is measured by the ability to elicit a full medical history, to diagnose a problem accurately, and to empower patients to participate in their own care. Empathy is not just about the appearance of competence but the reality of competent doctoring.

We end this section on empathy with the testimony of a patient about an exceptional clinician, which highlights the way empathy can be nested in a variety of other skills, such as listening, attentiveness, warmth, and trust. The payoff in terms of better patient care is evident.

> Yes, Dr. Jasper's ability is also a really good ability to listen and to empathize. He's really terrific at that, I consider him a friend, and when I go, we talk about other things [other than the illness] and there are times when I actually feel closer to him than to other people because I can say things to him that I wouldn't to my other practitioners.

Compassion

> *Compassion is the basis of morality.*—Arthur Schopenhauer, *The World as Will and Presentation*

We examine the trait of compassion last because it is a culminating response, grounded in empathy and giving more precise form to caring. We begin with a remarkable account of a patient's meeting with his clinician after a failed intervention, for which both patient and doctor had had high hopes.

> I: How did he respond to your coming back to his office? Your feet were now moving, but the pain had returned. He had done the surgery and your situation hadn't improved. How did he respond to that?
>
> R: He was very sad. I sensed he was grieving for me. I mean he wasn't simply feeling bad that things hadn't gone well. He was grieving for me.

Medical interventions run along a broad scale of success and failure. Sometimes patients are helped dramatically and sometimes only modestly. Occasionally patients emerge from treatment regimens unchanged. And, regrettably, some patients are worse off than before their treatments began. In this unfortunate case, mingled with the sense of regret over a failed procedure, this patient and his spouse found a feeling of deep appreciation for the fact that their clinician's grief was a grief *for* them. It was not just professional disappointment over an ineffective intervention, but a manifestation of true compassion.

Another patient described a meeting with the doctor after a major surgery to correct a chronic and debilitating sinus problem. This was the second surgery her clinician had attempted, and neither had been of much help to the patient.

> He was my sinus doctor. One of the most touching times I have had with a doctor was with him after he had to go into my frontal sinuses, which means he had to cut my head open.... And that was the second surgery he had done on me, so I had seen him a lot, and I remember I said to him: "Do you think I'm so emotional and sad and depressed and tired because of the surgery?" And he literally laid his head on his hands and cried, and he said, "If I could cure you I would." And you know, I'd never had a doctor tear up with me.

What is noteworthy here is that the patient sees the clinician is moved, literally moved to tears, and she remembers it as something exceptional and deeply caring.

There is a good reason why compassion is a central virtue in every major Eastern and Western religious tradition. Compassion is an expression of love. The English word "compassion" has its etymological roots in Greek and Latin, meaning "to suffer together with." Compassion is not just suffering recognized, but shared. It extends beyond emotional mirroring or empathic understanding. Compassion issues in responses intended to help and heal. Sometimes the responses are in words, as the scenario above illustrates. And sometimes they are deeds. The Hebrew Bible compares the compassion of

God to the compassion of a mother for her child and stresses its connection to actions of pitying, forgiving, and showing mercy. In the Christian Bible Jesus answers a question about who is one's neighbor through the parable of the "Good Samaritan;" the parable depicts a wounded man who is neglected by religious leaders who ignore him on the road; a stranger passes by and helps the man. The moral key to the parable is that the Samaritan helps the man because he is "moved by compassion."[14] Most chapters of the Quran begin with the verse, "In the name of God, the Compassionate, the Merciful." But perhaps in no tradition is compassion more central than it is in Buddhism. A familiar story is told that when asked by his personal attendant Ananda, "Would it be true to say that the cultivation of loving kindness and compassion is part of our practice?" the Buddha answered, "It would be true to say that the cultivation of loving kindness and compassion is all of our practice."[15]

One reason compassion is so prized is that it bespeaks a high level of moral maturity, one that is striking and memorable when displayed by clinicians. William Osler commended it unequivocally. "The practice of medicine is an art...a calling in which your heart will be exercised equally with your head."[16]

There is a recognition of common vulnerability in acts of compassion: "That person could have been me!" Clinical compassion is a morally mature expression of what in its earlier forms is general benevolence. As such, compassion is not a given. One cannot be sure it will be learned through common childhood experiences, or in the training of healthcare professionals. It does not automatically develop from honing skills of empathy. Acquiring it must be intentional. Patients, when vulnerable, are keenly aware of its absence and its presence.

SUMMARY

Holding a space for the patient's healing means creating a safe and receptive container, an "envelope" for clinical interaction. Building on reports of our patient informants, we have given a place of promi-nence in our analysis to bodily rapport, in both its spatial dynam-ics and its temporal rhythms. The clinician traits we have discussed throughout this chapter come to life within that clinical space. The most important of these traits to our patients were caring, empathic discernment, and compassionate responsiveness. In the absence of this essential set of abilities and traits, clinicians and patients cannot hope to work together effectively.

As we saw in chapter 1, being a patient first involves establishing a relationship with a clinician. Partnerships form around the inten-tion to care for the vulnerable body. We have argued in this chapter that the ability to hold clinical space is a precondition for develop-ing therapeutic relationships. The clinician traits we have discussed throughout this chapter can flourish within that clinical space. But where there is vulnerability and the possibility for healing there is also the risk of inadequate care, further wounding, and even aban-donment. In the next chapter, we offer detailed examination of how healing can be obstructed.

[3]

FALSE STARTS AND
FREQUENT FAILURES

Relationships with clinicians can be healing, but they can also be harmful. Among all the inspiring things we heard, we also listened to stories of some less-than-exemplary behaviors and practices that resulted in therapeutic failures, episodes that at their worst defeated any possibility for healing and left lasting psychic scars. In our 55 interviews there was a wide range of these negative encounters. Their scope encompassed both trivial and traumatic exchanges, extending from simple failures in communication because of jargon to insulting remarks, negligence, and, in a few cases, abandonment.

We recount some of these conversations for three reasons. The first is that such reports were not uncommon. While we began our interviews with an invitation for patients to speak about their relationship(s) with their current health provider(s), we also asked about other providers they may have seen. Because most of our informants, even the younger ones in our sample, had chronic conditions, they usually had experiences with many practitioners. As a result we heard a great deal about relationships patients perceived as the best *and* as the worst, as well as many in between these extremes. Second, we want to be true to the interviewees themselves, to honor what we have learned by recounting faithfully the narratives they entrusted to us. We hope that a candid recounting of both the good and the bad will help patient-readers become more alert to the possibilities, and that clinician-readers will self-consciously seek to avoid these common, but often inadvertent, relational pitfalls. Finally, retelling these stories of things gone wrong seemed to have a cathartic quality for our interviewees, especially when physical—or more often dignitary—injury resulted, especially if it occurred at a critical point in their illness experience, or during a moment of heightened vulnerability.

We call this chapter "false starts" because frequently the thing that doomed the relationship happened at or near the beginning, usually in the first session with the clinician. In a track meet a false start can sometimes eliminate the runner from contention before the race ever begins. When clinicians make false starts they sometimes eliminate the opportunity for a healing relationship to develop. Some adept clinicians can recover from early missteps, but in the stories we were told patients often did not provide an opportunity for clinicians to regain their footing or the patient's trust. We chose "frequent failures" as part of the chapter title to signal that our primary focus will be on the problems our informants discussed most often.

It should also be noted that these reports do not come from "bad" or "problem" patients. Such normative labeling is always precarious and loaded with assumptions that need unpacking. "Bad" for what? A "problem" for whom? All of us can be problem patients occasionally, and the likelihood for this increases when we are under stress. The persons we interviewed were for the most part selected for us by clinicians who had themselves been interviewed for our previous study. So while not all were "model" patients, in terms of always adhering to recommendations or treatments, it was clear that their willingness to talk with us was in part because they had productive, trusting interactions with the referring practitioner.

A review of our coding scheme for the interview transcripts may be helpful here, both in terms of the taxonomy we used to code negative clinician traits, and the number of interviewees who spoke of these traits. This book is mostly about relationships that work, and as we progressed, we began to collect and categorize the negative experiences with a few simple codes for failures. Yet the more we listened, the more complex the codes became as we sought to capture the details of why and how things go wrong. The results are reflected in table 3.1, which includes the complete coding scheme for negative

Table 3.1 NEGATIVE CLINICIAN TRAITS

Clinician Traits	Frequency
Poor communication*	32
Patient as object or number	31
Practitioner as incompetent or unprepared	28
Rushed practitioner	23
Inattentive	19
Negative body language	16
Inappropriate comments	15
Distracted	12
Provider discomfort	12
Arrogance	11
Avoided emotion	11
Jargon	11
Negative touch	7
Dishonesty	3
Paternalistic demeanor	1

* "Poor communication" served as a depository for a wide range of mistakes and misfires. For example, one patient said of her doctor, "He was a mumbler."

traits. The frequency associated with each negative trait represents the number of our patient informants who discussed this trait as something they had experienced. For example, "arrogance" was noted by 11 of our interviewees while 23 of the 58 discussed having been treated by a "rushed practitioner." Yet while this gives a sense of the frequency, with "patient as object or number" among the most often cited problems, frequency counts do not indicate the depth or quality of the negative experience for any particular patient. So we are careful not to suggest that being treated as an object or number is necessarily a more important problem than arrogance, but simply that it was discussed more often. Indeed, arrogance may have been a larger stumbling block for developing a patient's trust, depending on the contextual features of the specific interaction, the expectations of the patient involved, as well as many other factors. Our claim is that frequency does have some significance as an indication of the number of patients for whom this negative feature of the relationship stayed in their memories and was included in their narration about their providers. That this unwelcome feature is still a part of many patients' doctor stories, often years after the event occurred, is some measure of its importance. With these caveats in mind we seek to address the most frequently mentioned problems that this group of patients saw in their provider interactions, but we will also discuss some interactions that seem to have deeper meaning, even if they did not occur to the majority of our storytellers.

FALSE STARTS

He was either going to slow down and listen to me or we weren't going to continue.

Occasionally the first visit with a clinician leaves the impression with a patient that the relationship has important therapeutic value. One patient said, upon leaving the first appointment, "I remember thinking: she gets me. She sees I am a complex person. She was able to give me an immediate sense that I was supported." But regrettably, sometimes it only takes a moment for a patient to realize that the clinician can't really help. The following exchange is vivid testimony to an encounter that had no chance of having any healing potential. This excerpt comes from a patient who had been shot in the face and was seeking help for chronic pain several weeks after the surgery to repair her wounds.

I: So you knew almost immediately that this was not a doctor who could help you?

R: No absolutely; he was either going to slow down and listen to me or we weren't going to continue. I mean he had just told

> them he would meet them at 9. Well if you're going to meet
> somebody at 9, that's the 9th hole of a golf course. I've been
> shot; I'm not stupid.
>
> I: You heard him say that to somebody on the phone?
>
> R: On the phone, yeah, because he answered his phone while
> I was sitting there. And I'm thinking he did not answer that
> phone with me sitting there, but he did.

One interesting and understudied facet of healing is the environment, both the physical and the human environment, that surrounds the practitioner. One patient who uses a wheelchair spoke eloquently about the misfires that occur before the clinician even enters the picture.

> I'm amazed at how wheelchair unfriendly Dr. Stout's office is. I've
> had to change internists because it's just too hard to get to her
> office. And the receptionist... I mean their demeanor is so impor-
> tant and when they're snotty or snobby or you can't get their
> attention because they are talking to their boyfriend, or they've
> got three-inch fingernails that are dirty, and you're thinking, I'm
> at the chemotherapy center...

Perhaps cancer patients are more susceptible to false starts, missteps at the beginning of a relationship, than are patients with other diseases. The following excerpt was taken from an interview with a cancer patient who had an initial diagnosis of pancreatic cancer and had been referred to a regional center for evaluation.

> I went to the [Cancer] Center and let them look this over. And they
> wanted to go in and remove the tumor. They said they wouldn't
> get all the diseased tissue, so I would still have to have radiation
> and chemotherapy. I felt they were a little pushy. Maybe they
> weren't, but you drop a bomb on me.... I said I've got to go home
> and pray about this and think about it. They said, "We've got to

get you scheduled," and I said no. So we left there and we were supposed to have been back at 3:00 that afternoon. My daughter said, "What do you want to do?" I said, "I'm going home." And she called and told them I wasn't coming back. They were just hurrying up to get that knife out. I'm sure they're good doctors, and they thought they were doing what's best, but when you drop a bomb on a man, it's got to set there for a little while. I told them, "I can't make a split-second decision on this."

This patient subsequently decided not to return for treatment and at the time of the interview was enrolled in a hospice program.

FREQUENT FAILURES

The Patient as Object or Number

For doctors I'm just a series of parts.

Practitioners, insurers, and payers all tend to see the electronic medical record as a major advance in the quality of health care. The patients we talked to were less enthusiastic and many had comments on how the use of the computer during the office visit made the interaction seem less personal because it directed the clinician's attention away from the patient.

I think I felt, not neglected, don't misunderstand me, maybe cheated, when Medicare decided these physicians would all have their visits computerized. I think this took away from the personal relationship that one could have. We lost it then, when the doctor would come in and shake your hand and have a computer in the other hand. Everything was on the computer. You figure it doesn't go in through their ears or land in their head—it's on the computer.

Another patient, when asked about his relationship with a specialist she was seeing, said:

> R: I've never felt as close to Dr. Moore (neurologist) as I have to Dr. Hall (cardiologist), and I think one of the reasons—I think Dr. Moore is very competent—but he spends all the time I'm with him typing on the damn computer.
>
> I: Does he have his back to you, or is he positioned in some other way?
>
> R: I'm sitting there and he's typing, and what I'm really looking at is his left arm.
>
> I: His left arm, maybe not his best feature.

Generally specialists received the most criticism from our informants. One patient described his surgeon in terms both of his gratitude for the surgeon's technical skill and his disappointment about the surgeon's very limited interpersonal skills.

> So I'm pretty thankful, I mean he's one of the best in town. And he did a hell of a job. But zero bedside manner. Zero. He's like an accountant. No "How are you feeling? How's your back?" It's looking at the chart and talking in percentages as to whether or not he puts me under the knife. But zero about physical therapy or pain management. Zero ability to diagnose where the pain might be coming from, or interest in diagnosing that.

One of the interesting things to note about the patient's overall assessment is that because the physician did not talk about alternatives, the patient assumed that this physician was unaware of them. Lack of interest is taken as a deficit in the clinician's knowledge. This patient did undergo the surgery and was helped by it, but the lingering doubts about alternatives to surgery were still present in the patient's story of his care.

The clinician skipping over the introductory rituals for engagement, with a laser focus on the specialist's area of expertise, was a repeated theme in our interviews. Such a move ignores the patient's need to engage the clinician with their understanding of what is happening, which is sometimes key to the healing process and even to locating the correct diagnosis and finding the best treatment. One patient said her encounter with the practitioner was so "solution driven" that "I felt like I was part of a business plan." By contrast, this patient described her current provider as "attending to her patients on every level."

Many patients who spoke with us provided reminders about how simple the remedy for depersonalized communication may be, and how lack of skill in this area can turn potentially therapeutic encounters into the experience of being objectified. This patient had switched from conventional medicine to an alternative practitioner.

> I don't go to gynecologists anymore.... I just didn't feel like I was listened to. Because for doctors I'm just a series of parts, and "Let me give you what this part needs." I don't know when I've had a traditional doctor talk to me about what's going on in my life. It's just "What's your symptom," and "Let's deal with your symptom."

Finally, an especially reflective patient who has seen multiple physicians since early childhood relates how she learned to communicate her symptoms in a detached manner in order to put her doctors at ease.

> I had the best relationships with them if I spoke in medical jargon about myself. I spoke about my body as if it were somebody else's body, using medical language... sort of like a robot myself as I'm reporting what's going on with me. And I found, wow, this is a really good way to relate to these doctors because they seem much less cold and hard if I meet them in their own place; it then becomes the two of us talking about this problem.

This passage is remarkable in several ways. First it exhibits a self-conscious communication strategy after several failed attempts to establish common ground on the patient's terms. It also provides insights into how to get some partnership in the care. But at what a price! Certainly, it is a good thing for patients to be able to consider physicians' points of view, to learn the appropriate language for their condition, and thereby better identify with the treatment plan that is being offered. But adopting the clinician's perspective just to make the relationship less cold or to make the provider more comfortable is asking too much, especially when the patient is worried or anxious about their diagnosis. Also, objectifying oneself as a strategy for mitigating the ill effects of the provider's impersonal approach means relinquishing the need for simple recognition as a person that is absolutely necessary in human interactions. That such a strategy was adopted by this patient when she was a child speaks volumes about the vulnerability of children when seeking medical care for chronic conditions.

The Rushed Practitioner

They just want to get you in and out of there.

Closely related to objectification is the sense of being rushed through a medical encounter. One patient with a wide range of problems described it like this:

> So, I'd see the hypertension doctor for this. Then I'd see the neurologist for this. I ended up over the four years having 19 medications I took daily and I had 21 different medical specialists, and I was worse than ever; I was given the opportunity to take a total disability if I wanted to. So it was pretty alarming.... The system was finely tuned and all that was great, but none of them ever really touched me, talked to me for more than two or three minutes—rushed in, rushed out, rushed in, rushed out—or looked at me as a whole person. I was always this guy with hypertension, the guy with high blood sugar, the guy who gets the swallow test.

The patient continues:

> One of the things that puts me off is when the doctor doesn't
> want to hear a lot of questions, when they sort of blow you off,
> or they're in a rush. They don't have time to really talk to you.
> I know I'm not their only appointment that day, but there are
> questions. And they feel like any question you ask is kind of
> interfering with their time.

One of the findings from our interviews is how the experience of
being rushed works as a disincentive for follow-up visits, and the dis-
continuity in care that results. The following remarks are indicative
of many similar remarks.

> You know, I had a vasectomy. The doctor who did my vasectomy,
> he was just, get this thing done. No common touch; no "This is
> how you're going to feel"; no "Do you understand what we're
> doing here?" None of that. The doctors who always seem to be in
> a hurry, that have no patience, they just want to get you in and
> out of there, that doesn't do anything for me. It's probably one
> of the reasons I've gone for years and years and years without
> seeing a doctor.

Another patient put it this way when describing her therapist:
"He had really lousy bedside manner, and I think this conditioned my
response. Most doctors just don't have the time." Patients were also
insightful about the qualitative dimension of time, understanding
that it isn't so much about the minutes expended, as it is about the
quality of the interaction within whatever time is available.

> If the time [the clinician has for a patient] is reduced from 15
> minutes to 7 minutes, well it's like driving a car at the speed limit
> going to a meeting and you're gripping [the wheel] hard and
> anxious. You're going as fast as you can; you might as well relax
> and enjoy the scenery. Well same with a clinician who comes in

having to crunch down to 7 minutes—a breath, a smile, a "How are you?" and maybe we need to compact our visit a little today. So let's stick with what's really important. Almost everything can be accomplished in those 7 minutes if the clinician is calm instead of anxious, and exudes that to the patient who will stop feeling anxious about not having enough time. I don't recommend 7 minutes all the time. But sometimes it's inevitable. [It's] being in charge of what's going on, being in the space, being present.

The Inattentive Practitioner

He doesn't give me the feeling that he really cares about me.

Some relationships fail because the clinician is inattentive, usually not just on one occasion, but routinely and habitually. One of the most basic forms of inattentiveness is simply not listening. Typically portrayed as a simple thing to do, listening actually takes energy and concentration. It is a way of focusing or giving attention, and it always says to patients, "You are worth my time. I think this interaction with you is important. I am willing and able to be with you rather than somewhere else." All of us are skilled at recognizing this, even in this age of multitasking and efficiency. Fortunately, studies of multitasking have begun to show that it is quite inefficient, and that multitaskers often overrate their ability to do it.[1] Of course, the stakes are higher in healthcare interactions. People's well-being and even their lives can be determined by that level of attention. A positive therapeutic dynamic is ruled out immediately if either party is mentally absent.

The following scene illustrates the importance not only of paying attention, but also providing cues that one is paying attention. This interview was given with the patient and a friend of the patient (R2) present; the friend also knew the clinician being discussed. The message this patient wanted to convey is signaled from the beginning of this segment of the interview, then the friend and the interviewer get sidetracked, but the patient repeats the important message for emphasis—that inattentiveness signals the absence of care.

R: He gives you the impression he doesn't care.

R2: Dr. Snow you mean?

I: And how does he give you that impression?

R: He doesn't listen to you talking. Well, that's how I felt.

R2: It's something you pick up.

I: You can tell when you're not being listened to, body language perhaps . . . or maybe they have good body language but they're not hearing the meaning?

R2: They're listening to the words, but the nuances are not getting through?

R: He doesn't give me the feeling that he really cares about me.

Sometimes inattentiveness is a simple function of the clinician being preoccupied, or overwhelmed. Whatever the reason, the results are the same.

It was like talking to a robot. He never made eye contact the entire time. He was all business, shuffling papers. . . . I mean it was an impersonal thing. And it hurt like hell. Well, how do you put it? You almost felt like you were bothering him, and that you were putting him out, or that maybe you were exaggerating, or that it wasn't as big a problem as you might think.

One of the noteworthy things in this narration of the encounter is how—in the absence of any signals from the clinician that he is listening—the patient doesn't know what to think, but all the possibilities he conjures up are negative. And of all the forms of inattentiveness, having one's immediate pain ignored or minimized is one of the most distressing.

Setting aside for the moment the lost therapeutic potential of relationships, lack of attention can also lead to inferior care by conveying inaccurate information and discontinuing care. Here again there was a third party in the interview, in this case the patient's spouse (R2), who describes the frustration of a wrong diagnosis caused by inattentiveness.

R: I had one doctor, Dr. Davis, I felt never listened to me. He was just doing what he wanted no matter... and for that reason I had some problems with medication.

I: How do you know he wasn't listening?

R: You can just tell.

R2: He was treating her for things she didn't have.

R: And he would be very insistent on treating me for something that Dr. Billings had said not to do. And I said, "Well if you don't believe me call Dr. Billings, because this is what I was told."

R2: Dr. Davis told her she was diabetic. And she had this blood work done once a month and it had never been high.

R: Well it was high on certain medications; the medication will make it high.

R2: We finally convinced him Dr. Davis of that.

R: We finally convinced him that if he would look at the A1c... [the A1c, or HbA1c, is a form of hemoglobin that can be separated and tested as a marker of average blood glucose levels over the previous months prior to measurement].

R2: Cause her A1c came back normal.

R: I'm fine.

R2: And this finally convinced him, and he did the blood work and it came back normal, but it became a problem because Dr. Davis had classified her as diabetic and her insurance—Medicare's sending her all this stuff about diabetes, saying you have to get this...

I: And his not listening triggered all this?

R2: You know his not listening triggered them saying, as she entered the hospital, "Oh, you're diabetic," and her saying, "I'm not diabetic," and we had to go through a lot of hoops to get that taken off as far as her Medicare was concerned. They had her classified and were going to have to do all those extra tests, because she was classified as a diabetic when she was not.

R: They kept saying, "But you're not taking your diabetes medicine." And I said I'm aware that I'm not, because I'm not diabetic. Then they would say, "but you are diabetic." I said, "Well, I'm really not."

R2: And it was all based on that one visit. And you're saying to yourself, OK, one visit does not a relationship make...and if that doctor had truly been listening to her you would think he would have had her back in several times, he would have checked the blood work several times.... one panel does not make a person diabetic.

Clearly one visit can be enough to doom a relationship.

Sometimes tales of inattentiveness mean, very straightforwardly, that the clinician simply did not show up. The following patient describes an illness episode in which, for whatever reason, her primary care physician does not check in on her, or at least not in a way that she is aware of. Note the way this absence takes on a kind of indignity committed against her.

I think that's what shocked me, that I could be there [in the hospital] 49 days and my doctor didn't even come by. I think that's what you come to expect from a doctor. I'm a person.

It is noteworthy that this may not be a problem of inattentiveness in the way the patient thinks. It could be a failure to tell the patient that while in the hospital a specialist or hospitalist would be her primary doctor. For many older patients this runs counter to their expectations, and for many others it means a transfer of trust that may not be simple or feasible. After all, each new practitioner on the scene has to convince the patient of their capacity and willingness to help them and the dynamic of vulnerability and responsiveness must be engaged.

Finally, the following is an instance of inattentiveness that is relieved by a renewed interest in the patient when she needs a post-surgical procedure to resolve her problem.

She did not seem to care or be interested in me at all until about 10 days after the surgery. I was in the hospital for two weeks, and about 10 days after my mastectomies she came into the room, knelt on the floor, and herself drew out the fluid that was building up.... That was so caring of her, to come in and do that herself. It just broke the ice and I realized she cared and the relationship became better.

Avoiding Emotion

Brilliant man, [but] it's all technical . . . as a person, he's not there.

The role of the emotions in health care is much debated and frequently misunderstood. In the past the norms of medicine dictated tight emotional control for the practitioner, lest the capacity for rational judgments be compromised. Indeed, the traditional prohibition on treating members of one's own family is grounded in the notion that such a clinician would have too much emotional attachment to be objective and as a result was likely to render inferior care. More recently this norm of emotional "detachment" and its Cartesian assumptions have been challenged, and the higher wisdom is that affective distancing can be as debilitating as emotional over-involvement. The psychiatrist-philosopher Jodi Halpern describes what she believes is the appropriate balance and affective accuracy for appropriate emotional involvement in her book *From Detached Concern to Empathy.*[2] Physician-writer Jerome Groopman gives vivid testimony to the cost of emotional detachment in terms of medical mismanagement. When the affective sensibilities of the clinician are not engaged, less attention is given to patients and their presentation of symptoms and misdiagnoses are more likely to occur.[3] Still, for our patient interviewees, emotional distancing was very much in evidence and frequently cited as a barrier to building healing alliances with clinicians.

Sometimes the detachment can be understandable, even if not desirable. One patient spoke of her interaction with a transplant surgeon in terms that could excuse his behavior, even when she found it abrupt and callous. This perhaps indicates that putting oneself in the clinician's shoes may help to excuse the behaviors, but does little to remedy the lost possibilities for a more solid therapeutic alliance.

> There wasn't any doctor that understood [what the patient was going through]....When I met the heart and lung transplant surgeon, he just came in and looked at me, he didn't want to get to know me.... They don't want to get to know you because their patients die. He said, "I don't want to get to know you, I'm not your friend, but I will transplant you as your death occurs." And then he walks out.

One of the most interesting ways of avoiding genuine emotional contact with patients occurs when the clinician cloaks affective responses to the patient behind a veil of unremitting optimism. While optimism can be a very desirable trait in clinicians, sometimes activating a patient's expectancy for improvement,[4] optimism that is adamant or unqualified can come across as disingenuous and a shield against emotional honesty and availability. This patient discusses her discomfort with a doctor she was initially assigned.

> She's a little relentlessly upbeat for me.... It's not like she isn't listening, I think she is, and I think she's really taking good care of me, but sometimes she'll look at my chart and she'll say, "Compared to some other people who come in here you are doing so well." All my blood work is "great," and she uses the term "gorgeous" a lot..."Your cholesterol's gorgeous, your blood pressure's gorgeous." So at the end I sometimes say, "Then why do I feel like this?"

Interestingly, this patient stayed with this clinician despite her discomfort because she thought it was the best she could do, and "of all the doctors I have had, she is the most thorough."

The following is a poignant example of a clinician who avoids emotional contact by exiting immediately after delivering a devastating diagnosis.

> We used to spend our summers in Florida. I knew she [the wife] was getting more and more forgetful, and [had] various other

symptoms. And I thought, I want to find out what she has if I can so I can prepare for the future. So I went to a neurologist and he ran a brain scan on her…and a week later we went back to his office and he showed us on the screen all the stuff that was going on in her brain. It looked like it was mostly dead. It was an awful thing. And he said: "She has Alzheimer's. There's not a thing I can do about it." And I didn't plan to be a regular patient there or anything, but I felt it was the most awful put-down and put-off. He said, "There's not a thing I can do about it. Good bye." Here's some horrible news. And I think he was completely honest with me. But the way he put it. It was a disappointment.

This vignette illustrates tragic news compounded with the emotional equivalent of abandonment, all in the service of telling the truth. Many clinicians condemn this practice of "truth dumping," a practice that leaves the patient and family with devastating information but no help dealing with it. No suggestions about Alzheimer's support groups or encouragement about preparing the patient and family members for a radically changed life. No suggestion that although this will be tough, they might find they have the friends, family, or spiritual resources to make it bearable. When clinician responses are confined to the ability or inability to achieve a scientific fix, then the emotional elements necessary for healing are very likely thwarted.

Inappropriate Comments

The only thing he wants to know is if I have quit smoking.

Some comments are inappropriate anywhere, on any occasion. Many others are simply wrong for the context, ill-timed for the occasion, or offensive when left without explication, follow-up, or development. In our sample of patients we included 14 hospice patients, whose interviews were some of the most interesting and instructive. The following patient was interviewed in her own home about two weeks prior to her death. We entered the house for the interview at about 2:00 p.m. The patient was enjoying a gin and tonic and a cigarette.

She was still full of life, joyful, with an engaging sardonic wit and a self-deprecating sense of humor. One of her disappointments in her care arose from her interaction with specialists that she continued to see for various symptoms and quality-of-life issues. While her hospice care was excellent, her interaction with a pulmonologist was less than satisfactory.

> And going to my pulmonary guy, he just zones [out].... I could have sat there and lied to him [laughs]. You know it's depressing to go because there's not one positive thing coming out of him. He can't tell me anything that's helpful. And now I'm losing muscle tone. I can't believe I've got chicken skin [laughs]. And the only thing he wants to know is if I have quit smoking. Since I lost my husband I'm probably smoking more, but cigarettes is like hard dick, it's on every corner and it's always glad to see you. [laughs]

Later in this interview, she elaborates about a more general exchange not about inappropriate words but about inappropriate styles of communication in practitioners.

> You know, that's the one thing hospice doesn't do is lecture me. The visiting nurse is worried I'm gonna burn myself; she just asks me not to smoke with the [oxygen] hose up my nose. For fear of fire. But they don't lecture me on anything.

Another therapeutic misstep identified from our interviews concerned how a diagnosis was presented to a patient, not as a declaration of professional judgment, made deliberately and carefully, but as an afterthought, tossed in the patient's direction.

> I will never forget she was typing [the electronic medical record once more], her position at the keyboard was facing away from me. And she said, "I wonder if you have bipolar. Do you think you have bipolar?" And she looked at me at that point. [I said]

"Why are you talking like that? I didn't even think you were listening to me, and you're throwing that out.... Could you give me a little background on what you mean by that? I'm glad I got you to stop typing for a second, but really?" And I think that was one of the last times I saw her; I just thought she seemed very flippant about what was to me a very serious diagnosis.

The following exchange, inept because it was not contextualized or modulated by any understanding of the patient's life and history, or accompanied by any offer of help, as well as lacking in any reassurance, is brutal and accusational.

This neurologist I went to might as well have been from Mars. Well, he put me through all these tests, and then he said, "You seem to check out all right, but there's nothing you can do about this RLS [restless leg syndrome]; you're just going to have to learn to live with it." I said, "Well, you know it's coming from somewhere." He says "Yeah. But we don't know where, you're just going to have to learn to live with it." So he wasn't really helpful, after I had spent half a day with him.

What follows is an inappropriate comment in the context of a patient's fragile doubts about her potential for recovery. This interviewee was herself a healthcare professional. One of her own patients had been hospitalized, undergone surgery, and was not doing as well as expected during recovery.

I emphasize with the younger ones [the health professionals in training she teaches] to be very mindful of your words because they are very powerful. Many people in our culture give away all their power to the doctor. I tell them [patients], "No, you get to decide; you can say no at any point; you're not incarcerated. Why do you think you can't say no?"...The surgeons come in and they pull up your gown, there's no permission. I had this patient who was very depressed when I went in that morning.

She'd had abdominal surgery and she wasn't healing very well. It was a few days post-op, and she'd had a couple of setbacks and was just down in the dumps. And I kept emphasizing that whole day, you're getting better, and one day you'll look back on this [and say], "It was really difficult, but it's over and you'll move on in your life." She was having a hard time wrapping her brain around the fact that she would ever get out of the hospital…and she started to look better, and they brought her the lunch tray and she said, "I think I can eat this." I was so excited, we're making progress. The doctor came in, pulled back the tray, lifted up her gown, looked at her, and said, "You're not healing the way I would like," and left. She didn't want to eat after that; she was depressed and went one step forward, two steps back…. You don't lie to the patient, but you look for anything positive, saying, "Well, the swelling has gone down, your color looks better"; something to allow them to grasp on to. I know he wasn't aware of what he had done…. I was frustrated because there was nothing I could do after that. Anything I said—"Well everybody heals differently"—was hitting a wall; that was it. It didn't matter.

Harm to the patient, latent in many of the previous examples, is quite explicit here. Words can heal and words can inhibit healing.[5]

Finally, one patient we interviewed had a history of prostate trouble. The particular urologist the patient was seeing that day was not his usual physician, but his partner in the urology practice. The patient's wife was also present as the clinician entered the room, and it seemed to both the patient and his spouse that this clinician was completely unfamiliar with the patient's record. After questioning the patient about various tests and their results, the physician proceeded to the exam. This episode needs no commentary.

So he [the physician] says, "OK, you need to drop your pants." I said, "Well, my wife will step outside for this." And he replies, "I'm sure she's seen you naked before." And I said, "I just as soon she stepped outside." And he said [turning to the wife], "Well, if you want to, go ahead."

Negative Body Language

He will listen to the question as he's walking out the door.

We have already noted a variety of unwelcome body signals, including turning away from the patient, failure to make eye contact, failure to listen, appearing rushed or too busy for even elementary social exchanges, and other behaviors. We end with one more to underscore how powerful body language can be, and how very attuned to physical comportment we all are when we are patients. This example recounts an ophthalmology exam. Here, once again, the husband, who was the patient, and his wife are both present.

> R: He's like she [the patient's wife] says; he comes in, does his thing, and he goes out. And if you don't catch him...
> R2: Well, Tom [the patient] yelled at him one day. He said, "I have a question."
> R: Yeah. I'm not through yet. [laughs]
> R2: And yes he will listen to the question as he's walking out the door. [He's saying, in effect] "It better be a good one." It's difficult getting your questions answered unless you're ready to tackle him before he gets out of the examining room.

Another patient put it succinctly: "I would say to them [physicians]: 'If you get too busy to look at your patients, then you are too busy to have a patient.'"

One of the most notable things about this list of failures, misfires, and mistakes is that most—if not all—can be avoided. They are all essentially ways in which the patient is pushed into the background, sometimes in a direct and wholesale way, but often with small slights and off-hand gestures of disrespect that can be easily avoided.

However, the remedy is only in part a mindful rehabituation of clinicians, a learning of new habits and gestures, and a discarding of maladaptive ones through techniques of behavioral modification. The real agenda is one of recalling the common courtesies that one learned as a child and developing an attitude that truly does put the patient first. Such an attitude "shows." Patients are exquisitely sensitive to those who are only acting at being interested. In *Healers* we recounted the experience of a physician who as a resident had the opportunity to work with a famous psychiatrist who taught behavioral techniques to establish better interaction, giving instructions such as "Keep eye contact"; "Nod your head when the patient speaks"; and "Lean forward in your seat to show interest." The physician, then a resident, responded, "Wouldn't it be better to just be interested in your patients?"[6]

[4]

THREE JOURNEYS

In this chapter we have singled out three especially compelling interviews to present. We quote from considerable portions of each interview to allow the reader to experience the full flavor, impact, and import of the conversations we were privileged to participate in while doing this study. Here there is a chance to get accustomed to voices, to imagine faces, gestures.

To begin we will review what being a patient involves:

Table 4.1 BEING A PATIENT

Being a patient involves:
1) Relationship with a clinician
2) Shared intention to care for the health of the patient
3) Threat or reality of illness
4) Threat or reality of significant pain/suffering
5) The horizon of death (near or far)

A patient is a person who enters into a relationship with a clinician who is focused on the healing of the patient. Together these two engage in a series of activities designed to maintain health or recover balance in the midst of the full range of vulnerabilities that characterize living. In this chapter, we take a very close look at how three remarkable patients engage vulnerability and healing in their own lives, in partnership with equally remarkable practitioners.

There are three main reasons for offering extensive segments of these interviews:

1. Detailed accounts give us a chance to see, sometimes week-by-week, or month-by-month, the active process and concrete details of dealing with illness and health.
2. Interview accounts that span years or even decades give us a chance to observe the ebb and flow of illness and healing that shape a lifetime.
3. Extensive excerpts give us as readers and listeners a vivid picture of the personalities of these three patients and fascinating portraits of their primary clinicians.

The selections from the transcripts have been edited with the goals of continuity, clarity, and anonymity in mind. The intention is to give the reader maximum access to the interview itself.

The reader is, in a certain sense, about to enter into a conversation. It is a one-sided conversation, that is true. One person asks questions and listens. The other is invited to do most of the speaking. This of course fits with the purpose of our study and the role of patient interviews within that study. We urge you to resist falling into the mode of "hearing a story." Instead, think of yourself as the interviewer, silently taking part in the conversation. How would you have asked these questions? Think of yourself as the patient. How would you have answered some of these questions?

We do well to remind ourselves that such speaking and telling are part of a multifaceted process of incorporating one's illness into one's life-world, one's life story. And as such, they are virtually essential components in restoring wholeness. With that in mind, we ask you to listen actively: engage what is heard, support the speaker, witness the truth. This is what we tried to offer our interviewees—as part of a best practice for interviewing, yes—but also in appreciation for what they were sharing and what they continue to teach. We hope that at the end of each interview you will feel that you have met a person struggling with and trying to live well in often demanding situations.

These interviews contain themes the reader will already be familiar with: how patients build relationships with practitioners; how such relationships go awry; what kind of practitioners patients find easiest to build a relationship with; and how patients experience the clinical space skilled clinicians hold for them. But we have picked interviews that invite deeper exploration of three distinct types of patient experience: (1) that of a life shaped in its most minute detail by severe, chronic pain; (2) that of seeking out what today is called "alternative medicine"; and (3) that of finding wisdom and healing in the daily round of dying. Think of these explorations as being led by experienced guides—the patients.

There are common threads in the interviews. All three patients deal with a multiplicity of caregivers; each account gives prominence to "nonmedical" notions of healing; and there is the daily struggle to keep a healing space open in the face of enormous pressures. In the first interview, we see this happening primarily through love and recognition; in the second, stillness and balance; and in the third, friendship and candor.

One distinctive thing about this trio of interviews is that none of them, at first look, display the classic scenario of healing: feeling ill or getting injured; seeing a clinician; getting diagnosed and treated; going on with one's life. What we are presented with is one patient in debilitating chronic pain, a second patient whom most would consider essentially healthy, and a third patient dying of cancer. Healing is accomplished in radically different ways in each of their lives. But for each it is, finally, relationships that heal.

"IBUPROFEN AND LOVE"

As patients we are all now familiar with the clipboard in the waiting room as we check in to see the practitioner, asking about changes in insurance, current symptoms, weight loss, alterations in mood, and also now about the presence or absence of pain. Many of us remember when there were no smiling or frowning faces to circle to indicate levels of pain. The idea that pain is a healthcare "vital sign" is an important advance in care.[1] Yet, even so, physicians at various degrees of training routinely get more warning from their mentors about "drug seekers" than they do about the problems their patients can have when their chronic pain goes untreated.

For centuries medicine functioned under the oppressive dualistic legacy of René Descartes, the famed mathematician and philosopher, who confidently asserted that pain could be divided into two domains.[2] Physical pain was something derived from identifiable lesions of the body and channeled along neurological pathways to the brain; psychological pain was more dubious, and its modern heirs are medical suspicion and vigilance about malingering and "somaticizing." We are still in many ways functioning within a Cartesian metaphysics.

Chronic pain accounts for a large number of both healthcare visits and healthcare costs in the United States. Approximately one of every six people live with chronic pain, and pain is a major cause of adult disability. Such pain affects every aspect of the sufferer's life and can lead to the destruction of the human world, in severe cases overtaking the person's identity for both self and others.[3] The interview that follows shows us how this remarkable patient, with immense help from his spouse, and a treasured relationship with his urologist, makes his life work in spite of debilitating pain.

The pain of this patient was so severe that he stood for the entire interview. Although he was provided with the opportunity to stop and rest, or to end the interview, he persisted for two hours. This patient was roughly 60 at the time we spoke with him and was accompanied by his wife, who has been critical to his care. In the transcript, the patient is R1 and his spouse is R2. Dr. H is the urologist who is the primary focus of R1's comments. Dr. A is R1's back surgeon, and Dr. P is one of his primary care physicians.

I: Let's start with the beginning. Maybe you could tell me a little bit about how you decided to go see Dr. H. What were the circumstances?

R1: Back in the mid-90s, I had kidney stones, quite severe, and I was being treated very well by a physician, but a switch in insurance made it impossible for us to continue.... I was having lithotripsies [procedure to break up kidney stones] fairly often. I got a list of people who were on the new insurance plan and my current doctor recommended Dr. H. At the first meeting, Dr. H. right away established a rapport with me when he said he thought well of a colleague. He was self-effacing, and he wanted me to be very comfortable and that began our relationship. This was the "get-to-know-you" visit, for you to get to know me and to see if you want to work with me that's the way he phrased it—not if I want to work with you—but if you want to work with me.

He then looked at my X-ray and said, "Of course as you know, your back is a mess." And he said, "How do you live with this?" And I said, "Well, I have an extraordinary wife." And he said, "Well that's good, thank God for that." But he said, "From the looks of this, I wouldn't know how you live with this. But our job is to deal with the kidney stone issues and here's what we're going to do in the short term." He set a follow-up appointment for another X-ray, he wanted a time lapse scan. That was 17 years ago.

I: What helped you decide that he was somebody you were gonna work with?

R1: I don't want to minimize the professional side, but that was in combination with the personal side. He took me back and showed me the X-ray and talked in great detail about various things and helped me to understand. He acted like we both had almost unlimited time even though the day was ending. He took notes on what I said, he wasn't just asking a question and it was left floating in the air. He was writing down what I was saying. Very professional.

But the personal dimension only grew, and has only grown over the years to the point where I count him a dear friend. I would get there for my appointment and he'd say,

"I've got something I want you to see." He'd take me back to the inner sanctum, the *sanctum sanctorum,* and he'd show me a recent book or one that was classic that he enjoyed and if I knew the book, we'd talk about it a little bit. Sometimes he had a poem from some author that he really enjoyed and he had it copied and given to me. I took him a book occasionally or recommended one and he would get the book and then he would tell me about what he'd read and what had really impressed him. It was not simply stuck up on a box somewhere, he was looking at it, this is what he does, he's always doing this.

R2: And one time I couldn't be there and he helped undress Richard. He helped him get undressed.

R1: He undressed me, we did the procedure and then he dressed me again.

R2: And that's not a simple thing with his back condition.

R1: No and very carefully, carefully, not wanting to exacerbate.

I: So you felt comfortable with him doing that?

R1: Oh yes.

Being a patient is a particular form of remembering and expectation. It is joint memory and joint expectation, because shared with a practitioner. This sharing can be lived as a full partnership, as something bordering on friendship. Together they come to understand and respond to critical events that make vulnerability focal.

R1's back problems began as a result of a motor vehicle collision. Six weeks after the accident he went to an orthopedist complaining of back pain. The diagnosis was a herniated disk. To R1's surprise, the minor rear-end collision had caused damage that would change his life forever. The orthopedist offered him several options for treatment but R1 held off for several years.

R1: But I didn't have any of the treatments done because I was just getting started at the publishing house and there were very few jobs. But there were days I went to work that I was absolutely dazzled with pain and the woman who hired me knew it and she would let me do things, relax in various ways or pace or walk, work the way I needed to work. I also worked more hours because I realized I wasn't doing nearly what I thought was enough per hour. But I had to tell my assistant editor that I had a severe back problem because there were days I was so numb with pain I couldn't talk, but I could work. I lived on Ibuprofen and love basically.

R2: Didn't you go several years, Richard, without seeing anybody?

R1: Yes, I went on for years only seeing Dr. H very occasionally, I'd say about once every six to eight months. It started out more continuous, but the X-rays did not show at that point that the stones were getting worse. At that point if I had a urinary infection I went to my primary care physician, Dr. P.

R1: I'd always had some difficulty sitting, but in 2001 I got so I could hardly sit down at all and the pain in the neck had gotten worse. It had not dissipated and I knew I needed some help.

R1: Dr. P sent me to Dr. A, who has performed surgery on me five times. Dr. A calls three of those surgeries, "The most important three failed surgeries." Everything went right, the titanium is there, the fusion, the grafting of bone took place, the cervical one and lumbar one,

R2: But nothing helped.

R1: and they all failed in stopping the pain, but he went over everything with me in such detail ahead of time. Giving me the odds on everything. Now he is a quiet gentleman, you wouldn't think he was a doctor.

R2: Quiet and gentle.

Prior to surgery, R1 went through intensive physical therapy for six weeks to determine his level of function and potential for recovery with or without surgery.

R1: The physical therapists showed me the report. They actually gave me a copy of their report to Dr. A, after this six-week period. It said, "This man is in a great deal of pain. He is attempting to do what we try to do but he can't do it, he is bearing up in life. And we're quite convinced he has a herniated disc and probably both in the cervical area and in the lumbar area." Dr. A did a lot more tests and he found problems, a lot of problems here and a lot of problems there. He discussed both areas [cervical and lumbar], he discussed probabilities. I asked him which one should he do first? He said, "You have very severe problems in both areas, either one, the choice would be yours." He said, "They are equally severe and debilitating."

Well I chose the lumbar because that's the one that was keeping me from sitting down and I had these great dreams, I was going to return to work in October. But he told me the odds for about seven different outcomes. The worst outcome was death and there was a chance of that, and then the next worst outcome was that it would become worse and there was a slight chance of that. There was a little bit greater chance that the surgery would on the one hand succeed but not reduce the pain at all and then two or three other possibilities. The very largest one of course, 70 percent of the people, the surgery cured the problem. Well I had the surgery, and my wife tells me that when he came down to talk with her that morning while I was up in post-op, he told her, "I don't know how he's functioned?"

R2: "I don't know how this man's functioned. I don't know how he's worked; I don't know how he stands the pain."

R1: Yes, that's what he told my wife. I actually was pleased to hear that because I felt I wasn't being a wuss, I didn't want to be a wuss.

I: He was acknowledging your ability to endure great pain and function at a high level.

R2: Yes.

I: Because pain could be considered a subjective experience.

R1: Yes, yes. But the surgery took quite a bit longer than he thought it would take and he found more problems. He said to me, that it was the most complicated spinal surgery he had done, except for some oncology patients.

Much of the beauty of this patient's account is derived from the depth of sharing with his practitioners that he is able to convey. But there also are accounts of experiences that drive deeply into long-standing relationships between this patient and his family caregivers. As one would expect, there are moments specially charged by the intensity of illness and pain, as in the following account.

R1: I would just like to say,
  I: Go ahead.
R1: I had, do you mind me saying this?
R2: I don't know, what are you going to say?
R1: Something about us.
R2: What about us?
R1: We were able to make love one time.
R2: Yes, that's right.
R1: It was fantastic....it was fantastic, as it had been months since we had last made love. It was fantastic.
  I: This was after the surgery?
R1: Yes, this was October.

For this patient and his spouse, recollection and hope, dynamic and bodily as they are here, seen alongside the challenges of extraordinary pain, produced an extraordinary tenderness.

Three months after his initial lumbar surgery, R1 was encouraged by the improvements in his daily life. His horizon looked favorable.

R1: So I was on top of the world, back to work, my wife would drive me home at noon, I'd work from 9 to 12 and they arranged her schedule so she could do that, she works there too. I thought things are going to be so good, my neck was still bothering me, but I thought well, another year I'll have that surgery. Then on the second Monday I had worked my 3 hours, my wife took me home, I lied down on my bed and I started to doze off and all of a sudden I came to, something had shifted and I felt my legs moving again and I felt the pain increase and I wept. I went back to work the next day, but I couldn't bear it, my wife had to take me home. I went back to Dr. A.

I: He had done the surgery and your situation hadn't been improved, how did he respond to that?

R2: Very sad.

R1: He was very sad. I sensed he was grieving for me, he wasn't simply feeling badly that he hadn't done well, he was grieving for me. And he may have even put his hand on my shoulder and he said he was very sorry. We had some X-rays and the titanium was still holding, the vertebrae were in place, the suspension or the fusion seemed to be continuing to develop, they used some bone from me and some donor bone.

R2: But the nerve, the nerves were too damaged. Because the nerves did not heal. That's a lot of years in a great deal of pain.

After multiple surgeries, R1 continued to cope with intense pain and debilitation. He remembered a nurse practitioner from Dr. A's staff who was especially attentive to his daily world.

R1: And then the nurse practitioner who works with me and the pain pump is a dear friend too. I just love her.

I: What's amazing about her?

R2: She's very interested in him.

R1: She's interesting, she's funny, she's very concerned about me. She always makes suggestions, recommendations.

R2: Try this.

R1: And I had a period where I was falling. One time I fell and got a concussion and a chip on my chin. I had a face fall that was the worst one I ever had, worse than the concussion. I also had a bad fall here that my wife saw.

R2: I couldn't get to him fast enough,

R1: and I went backwards and hit the wall and went down and peeled the paint right off the door. The nurse practitioner demanded that I get help.

R2: "No more of these falls!" she said.

R1: "Yes, I'll [nurse practitioner] come to your house and make sure. I won't put anymore Dilaudid in your pain pump! You have got to get a walker."

R2: Five walkers.

R1: I have five walkers they do different things.

R2: But the nurse practitioner is always making suggestions, simple things to try to help. She's always giving practical advice you know.

R1: Yes, but also we have similar sense of humor and it's not an intellectual relationship, although I would say there is a, there was a sense of the sacred. I mean she is just remarkable and she is such a good person. But there is a sense of the sacred, we talk about God now and then. She is not an intellectual in that way, she's very smart, but she's very warm.

R2: She's family oriented.

R1: and very acute on practical issues and suggestions and notices if I'm limping more.

I: She's paying attention.

R1: She wants to know exactly, how long have you been limping like that? Or if I'm bending forward more, "How long have you been curving this way?" I have loss of my left hand. She presented that to Dr. A, they did a conductivity test and it was very bad. They did surgery on that at the NP's initiative, but the surgery again didn't work.

Noticing and responding to changes in our bodily world are the core activities of health care. Patients seek the help of healthcare professionals in hopes they can provide careful attention and practical, sometimes lifesaving, care plans.

I: Looking back now, what would you say were highlights that really define the relationship with your urologist, Dr. H?

R1: Well one of them was doing the cystoscopy and we talked about a book that I had recommended. He had read it and we started talking and there was an anesthesiologist there. I was gowned and bare butted and all the rest, I had already been placed on the surgical bed and he was standing next to my head and we were talking about this book. We were talking about the problems of translating, how do you translate what is so extraordinary in German into extraordinary English? And we were discussing a couple of Rilke's *Poems for the Hours*. He said, "They tell me we've got to get going here. So we have to put a hold on this, maybe you can think about it while you're under and we can talk about it a little bit later."

R2: And then not too long ago, it may have been the time he helped you when I was not there, he reached over and he said for Richard to take care of himself, he really loved him.

R1: Yes, he told me that. He put his hand on my arm, he said, "You're a good man Richard, I love you." He put his hand on my arm and told me he loved me. Yes, yes and I really love him too, he's remarkable, he's one of the finest human beings I've ever met and it has been my great good fortune that he has been my urologist and has gotten me through some dicey things.

The powerful currents of surrender and of intrusion and acceptance involved in being a patient tend to generate memories and hopes that have a startling body-intimacy—the kind of intimacy we most often have with partners, lovers, and family members.

R2: And there was the time he had an emergency where he couldn't urinate.

R1: And then I couldn't urinate at all and I called and told them I couldn't urinate and it was Dr. H's day off and he came in.

We did not have an anesthesiologist, so this was a painful one, he did a cystoscopy without anesthesiology. He had an assistant, but what they did basically was go up with a variety of tools into my urethra and up into the ureters—I think I'm getting the terms correct—and they scraped out stone fragments, as much as they possibly could. And stone after stone after stone came out and I could hear them hit the pail. He started out at the beginning, he said, "Richard, don't kick me, remember I'm trying to help you, don't kick me, if you're gonna kick, let me know." And I didn't kick. It was painful. They usually knock you out for that. But it was so blocked they had to do it immediately and they had no anesthesiologist, and I kept hearing the stones hit the pail. And every now and then he'd say, "Are you still with us? Can you take more?" And I'd say, "Yeah I can take some more." And he said, "I'm pretty sure I can get some more." I said, "Okay." And he kept working and working,

R2: This was on his day off.

R1: Yes, he came in with a suit on and just tossed his coat in a chair and got gowned and washed and prepped and in we went. I wasn't expecting any surgery or anything, but that's what we did and finally the pain became really tight and I was holding my legs and I let out a little laugh, I said, "That kick might be coming in another minute or two." He said, "Well, I've done almost as much as I can and I'm surprised you haven't killed me." He said, "If I were you, I'd have killed me."

In terms of general reflections, there was a time 2½ years ago. We lived in southeast Nashville, I loved the house we lived in...but we needed the kids a lot of times to do things for us and they were 42 miles away, but I loved that house and I didn't want to move. But my wife needed to move, I realized it was killing her, it was killing her and she is life to me. She's the greatest, she's the greatest proof of the existence of God to me and so for her sake, I consented that we would move over here.

R2: But he got very depressed.

R1: I just got very depressed here and I thought having gotten over here which is what my wife needed, the best thing I could do now would be to die, but I wouldn't commit suicide because she couldn't get any benefits, so I will just stop eating, so I stopped eating and I went from about 260 pounds and I think the lowest I got was

R2: 160? 170?

R1: 167 pounds. Yeah, they [R2 and R1's daughter] took me to see Dr. H.

R2: Oh, he about had a fit.

R1: Yeah, he sat there and talked to her and I was pretty lifeless but I could hear what they were saying and he said, "My God, he's dying, he is dying, you have got to do something." He said, "I can't save him as a urologist, we can solve certain problems here, but we've got to get a team together, we gotta get a nutritionist and we've got to get the neurologist, and I'll be on the team, we'll get the psychiatrist and your primary care physician will head this up, or we're going to lose him, because this is not going anywhere." Well my daughter started as a nurse and she's still an R.N. but she has a few more initials now. So she with Dr. H,

I: Organized a team?

R1: Yeah, because my primary care physician didn't respond. And that's when we dropped him. They got medicine that would make me, it would force me to eat and I begged them to not make me take it, I said I would start gradually eating again if they wouldn't make me take that medicine and so my daughter didn't make me take it. She said we'll give you a couple of days and we'll see and I started eating gradually again and I've gained back to where I'm just about the right weight.

R2: Dr. H made him realize that he still had life and that he was important to other people.

R1: He was so passionate in talking to her right in my presence, although not to me, but to her, that I realized he had an interest in me as a human being. I realized how much my daughter had an interest in me as a human being and I realized, I came to the conclusion my wife would be better off with me as a pain in the neck because you know we took each other for better or for worse and she got the "for worse" for years now.

R2: It's been great honey.

R1: It has been, it is, great.

R2: That has more to do with healing than anything.

R1: But Dr. H did that. I would be dead if he had not done that. So I have plenty of reason to love him and for him to tell me, "I love you, you're a good man," is one of the greatest honors I have ever been bestowed.

One of the many remarkable facets of this narrative is the healing power of being told that one's courage is noticed and admired. It is of course valuable to have one's family and friends take note, but to have one's virtues named by professional caregivers, who routinely see pain and how it is borne, has a special meaning. It is, as this patient says, "one of the greatest honors I have ever been bestowed."

Also evident here, among many other things, is the foundational nature of deep caregiver relationships for healing, for both professional and familial caregivers. Realizing that his family needs him, understanding that he is not better off dead, and that love sustains both him and his family, is transforming. His wife put it definitively in her closing remark: "[Love] has more to do with healing than anything."

A line from a letter Keats wrote in 1819 to his brother and sister-in-law, George and Georgiana Keats, could serve as an epigram for this interview: "Do you not see how necessary a world of pains and troubles is to school an intelligence and make it a soul?" That letter also contains a famous phrase that fits well with the chronic pain story of the patient interview above. Chafing against traditional religious understandings of life as a "vale of tears" to be followed by a life of bliss—which might fit our patient, but only partially and poorly—Keats insisted that life is better understood as a "vale of soul making."[4] According to this way of thinking souls are forged and acquire unique identities through the experiences they undergo and endure in this life. For Keats this was the mechanism of "salvation," what in more prosaic terms, we have entitled "healing." And it is this insight that is offered in this patient narrative, summarized in his final evaluation of his marriage and his life: "It has been, it is, great."

"STAYING TUNED UP"

The bulk of our interviews were done with patients of allopathic clinicians who were trained in the biomedical framework dominant in the Western world. The emphasis in this ubiquitous practice and education tends to be on diagnosis and treatment, couched in conventional scientific categories and aimed wherever possible at conventional biological remedies. In many life-threatening and emergency situations and with discrete physiological problems like a broken arm or a clogged artery, this is precisely what we want. But a noteworthy trend in health care over the last two decades has been the rapidly increasing numbers of patients augmenting biomedicine with visits to "complementary and alternative" (CAM) healthcare practitioners and choosing one of those practitioners to be their primary care provider.[5]

Twelve of our interviews were done with patients of CAM practitioners: acupuncturists, chiropractors, craniosacral therapists, and mindfulness therapists. We had several reasons for including this class of patients. First, because of this trend toward alternative medicine, we wanted to get a "fieldwork" sense of what these impressive numbers are about. Second, it is apparent from the literature that patients seek CAM clinicians because they work from healing philosophies that are more understandable and attractive to patients. Third, CAM practices include, as a routine matter, those which in a biomedical model tends to be labeled "wellness activities." This is a fascinating phenomenon, in and of itself. Fourth, we found the CAM practitioners we interviewed for *Healers* to have been unusually thoughtful about how they established healing relationships with their patients. Therefore, it only made sense to interview some of their patients.[6]

We have placed "complementary and alternative" (CAM) in quotation marks because there remain issues with this label and no small amount of bias. First, there is a question of precision. A wide range of healing practices and disciplines—themselves radically different from one another in terms of development, sophistication, experimental validation, and coherence—are being swept into the capacious bin indicated by "CAM." But far more important is the distorted picture we get of CAM practices when they are approached as isolated techniques. To give one example: The medical systems developed in China (acupuncture, herbal treatment, and Qigong) include carefully developed, systematic practices for diagnosis and treatment. There is, as well, an understanding of the body—a physiology—based on centuries of observation and trial and error. Traditional Chinese medicine in turn is nested within a comprehensive worldview distinctly different from the one implicit in modern Western biomedicine. We are not dealing with a menu of alternative modalities that can be plugged into biomedicine where biomedicine fails. Rather, these are whole systems of understanding what it means to be a human being in the world.

We have chosen the interview that follows in significant part because this patient articulates just these points so clearly. In it we see a patient continuing to develop her relationship with her practitioner, Mary, *as part of the ordinary rhythm of her life*. Rather than being driven by crisis intervention and "after-the-fact" care, the approach to healing this patient describes and explains turns away from the exceptional and the dramatic to emphasize the everyday. In just this sense, what is found here is a complete and radical alternative to our conventional biomedical practices.

I: How long have you been seeing Mary, and what was going on in your life at the time that you began to see her that made you think, "Time to find a practitioner"?

R: It has probably been not quite two years. She had been recommended to me almost 10 years ago by my Zen teacher.
I have a Zen meditation practice, and my teacher had gone to
see Mary over the years for a variety of things, and had recommended her, and, in fact, thought she would be very helpful,
and I didn't have anything acute enough to send me in that
direction until a couple of years ago.

I was facing a surgery at the same time I was under a tre-
mendous amount of stress because my sister had been diagnosed with breast cancer. Our mother had died of breast cancer
when she was 40. I have a sister who is two years younger
than I am, and they now offer genetic testing, if you've got
any family history. And after a lot of discussion, we decided to
go ahead and get the testing. She was positive. And then I got
tested, and I was positive also. So there was just this big storm
of stuff that I was going through. I was fearful for my sister. It
stirred up a lot of things in me, long held grief and anger, and
then, I also decided to have my ovaries out. That's the long
lead up to the surgery as a kind of a prophylactic measure, and
I have no disease, but I decided to do that.

I was into my first year of chairing the department, and I
couldn't take a medical leave. I just had to do the surgery and
go back to work. From what I had read about acupuncture,
also, I heard that many people benefited from being treated
before a procedure and then there were various physical manifestations of the stress that I thought she might help me with.
So, that's why I started seeing her.

I: What gave you the confidence to keep seeing her?

R: She really took the time to take a full history; and it was a different kind of medical history than the one I'm used to having
where you just send your records. This was more like, "Well,
let's just talk to me about what's going on," and it's been a
therapeutic kind of relationship in a way that is not just about
whatever physical ailment (*laughs*) I present, which I now
understand is more about what this kind of medicine is like.

I think of her less as an alternative medicine practitioner, she's more like a healer to me. I feel like I go to her for healing.

We always start by talking about what's been going on, and I have shared things with her that I would only share with a person that I felt close to, and would not normally come up and chit chat with a doctor. Most doctors, in my experience, just don't have the time and they're there to treat some part of you. I've had doctors inquire about me more generally, but, and I'm not finding fault with the doctors. It's just a different kind of relationship than I've ever had with somebody that was also trying to take care of me, body and mind, basically. That's part of why I have stayed. I began to realize that this would be a different kind of relationship.

In addition to a different way of thinking about and doing health care than allopathic medicine offers, many if not most CAM practices are run as small businesses. They tend not to be part of larger practitioner groups or hospital conglomerates. And they mostly operate outside of insurance and federal reimbursement programs. This allows these clinicians to shape their daily schedules and the details of care to suit their own styles, educational backgrounds, and philosophies of medicine and healing. These elements are immensely attractive for increasing numbers of people.

R: And I also think that I just liked her right away, and I can imagine that I might not have clicked with somebody else. Maybe I was preconditioned to like her because my Zen teacher recommended her, but I'm also capable of having independent judgment, I just felt like this was a person I wanted to see again, and so that's been a big part of the treatment I've received from her.

I also really appreciated that she explained a lot about what she was doing or what her principles were when she was operating. I appreciated that she had a background in Western medicine. So, she would understand where I was coming from, and that she also complemented acupuncture with her knowledge of Chinese medicine. She has given me things, for example, to help support various functions that I have found quite helpful. And when I got to the integrated medicine people,[7] the MD that I was working with, when I gave her the list of things that I'd been taking, she said, "Oh, this is great." And I showed her some particular formulation of a calcium compound, and she looked at the thing, "Oh, we don't," she said, "I've never seen this. This is fabulous." So all of these things gave me confidence, all this cross-checking, but I think that the main factor was that I really felt Mary's compassion. It was a kind of openness, and gentleness, and listening. There was a very deep listening that was expressed in how she treated me. Not just the listening, but also the kinds of things that she picked out, and then tried to attend to.

These details about this patient's visits to her acupuncturist are very helpful for seeing how CAM can fit into a plan for maintaining balance and wellness. Note also the range of "therapies" offered as the visit progresses.

Well, I really did not know what to expect. I'd heard a lot of people say that it really doesn't hurt, it's not something that hurts. But I was a little apprehensive. I don't like needles. In fact, the worst part of any procedure for me is a needle or stitches. And I think part of what made me feel comfortable about getting on the table is that you don't really have to strip to do it. It's not your standard exam. You're not in a gown, there's no curtain and they wait for you to get undressed. It's more like, "Well, why don't you hop up and relax." It was sort of an invitation to get comfortable, and she made sure I was comfortable. She put a bolster under the back of my knees, just was very careful to make sure that I was in a position that I felt supported in and comfortable in. She always asks if I'm warm enough. And she now knows me well enough to know that I don't have very good circulation in my feet, and so, at this point, that's something she doesn't even need to ask.

But she was also the person, I developed some arthritis in this joint, and she was the one that said, "You know, I really think it's arthritis," and to tell me, "A lot of women in menopause actually develop this," and I had to get an X-ray, finally, for my doctor to confirm it. So, I trust her instincts, and she just put me at ease that way. And also, the way she touched me was very sensitive, very gentle, and, clearly listening with more than her ears, listening with her fingers. And she will always tell me what she's doing. Like, "This point is good for this," or, "This point is called a thus and such point, and here's how it works." So I don't know that much about the meridians, but I appreciate that she's trying to explain to me why this needle in my foot is gonna help this other thing and how all of those are lined up. So, all of that made me feel, again, just very cared for and comfortable and not apprehensive about what was going to happen. I usually fall asleep as soon as she walks out the door to leave me for a few minutes.

And she has recommendations about food, too. She'll say, "This is a good time, given what's going on with you and the time of year, it would be good to try making this." She'll give me recipes. It's like a complete treatment, which is something that I find lacking elsewhere.

Before I started with Mary, I went to an integrated medicine practice in part because I wanted everything to be attended to under one roof. Before that, I had an endocrinologist over here and a gynecologist over there, but I never really felt like people were communicating very effectively—or that I was communicating with them very effectively. But now, with this integrative medicine group, everybody has access to all the records, so that sometimes my primary care physician will pass on feedback she's gotten from other team members about what I'm dealing with. Mary's doing that kind of integration within the tradition she works in, and that's something that I also really appreciate.

The intertwining of spiritual practice and teaching with therapies offered by this practitioner are a consistent theme in this interview. This is commonplace among CAM patients. The ease of building bridges with spiritual practice is for many a significant reason for seeing a CAM practitioner.

I: Are there ways that your work with Mary intersects with your Zen practice?

R: The tradition of Zen that I practice is Soto Zen. It's the San Francisco Zen Center, and in it there's no clear boundary between body and mind. And I, being the thoroughly Westernized, you know, twenty or twenty-first century with a lot of head consciousness, it's hard to understand that at first. And so, I think one thing that I really appreciate about this is that Chinese medicine tends to try to integrate in the same ways, and it's made me a lot more sensitive. I think the Zen practice plus this kind of treatment have just made me a lot more sensitive to that lack of boundary. The root of the teaching is, what you think is not your mind. But it took some kicks in the teeth to maybe fully embrace that, and it's a relief actually. (*laughs*) It's a big relief to be able to put down the thinking.

And I think the kind of constant noticing, that way Mary goes about sort of checking out my pulses is important. She's usually right, too, when she says, "Hmm, you're a little sluggish here." And it helps me too, it supports my awareness, that's the nonthinking awareness, I think. And I find that sometimes the effects of what she's done are pretty dramatic. I have this spasm in my back. It's between my shoulder blade and spine, and it cramps a lot. If that's bothering me, she puts needles in there. Boy, it's a really dramatic physical effect. It's what you would expect from medicine if you took a pill—it fixes it. It feels like it fixes it.

A lot of the other things she does are not fixes like that. It's more of a kind of rebalancing, and if I cannot just go back into my head after I leave her, and just try to let all of that sink in. I try to visit Mary later in the day so I can go home and not go back to work. It helps me to be aware of very subtle things in my overall general consciousness. So, I think they work together well, frankly. I make an appointment when I don't have a specific physical ailment, if I haven't seen her in a few weeks, I'll just make an appointment, and there's usually something going on otherwise, and I do it partly for the therapeutic relationship. I find her just very supportive, and there's usually something that needs tuning up. (*laughs*)

I: Anything in the last few visits that kind of epitomizes what your relationship with her is about or what she offers?

R: Well, I had an appointment in February, which I had to reschedule, and by the time I did see her, I was coming down with a bad cold that had a lot of the symptoms of the flu without the fever. And so I ended up really coming down with this, but what she did was keep me going for that week. She gave me this real sense, "Let me help you ward this thing off," and she knew I was really busy, but she just said, "If you don't have an hour or you don't have 45 minutes, come in, we can do something even in 20 minutes." And she gave me some mega Echinacea with goldenseal, and I just felt strengthened by all of that. And then when I called her next she said, "Oh, I can hear that it's got into your lungs, and, how're you doing?" I said, "Much better, but, why don't I come in," and so I saw her this past week. And I felt like she was driving out the last of it, 'cause I was still very tired, and finding it hard to stay with my regular schedule, not so much because I was still sick, but I just didn't seem to be able to get enough sleep.

This patient brings an unusual skill set to bear on her own health and development. She is able to move comfortably among various kinds of healthcare providers, with some appreciation for the strengths of each. And she is able to understand all of that activity in relation to her spiritual practice and her position as the chair of a university humanities department. Her range is as remarkable, in its own way, as her acupuncturist's is.

So, I also find that what she does frequently is just encourage doing what I know I need to do. One thing I've had to explain to my Zen teacher, and I try to break myself of actually, is that I think academics are so conditioned to ignore, to just push, push, push, push past fatigue, push past the point of no return, you'll sleep when you're dead, you know? Mary provides this kind of constant encouragement, "Are you sleeping? How's your sleep?" I've developed insomnia for the first time in my life. I used to sleep like a rock. Now, I wake up at, you know, two o'clock in the morning. But it's also menopause. I got plunged into a surgical menopause.

So, the other reason I've kept coming back to Mary is that, I was already entering menopause, but just like boom, I hit the wall, and as that has unfolded, it's like, who took over my body and what are they doing with it? So, she's really helped me with the symptoms, insomnia, various things that all of a sudden started to hurt that never hurt before. I have sometimes clung to her as somebody to check in with and to get a reality check. It's also a way to find some relief from all of this change. So in some ways I feel like the big changes are settling down, but she supports my taking care of myself during all the other hours and days of the week and month that I'm not there.

This is not the first or only time where she's said, "If you can even get in here for 20 minutes," or one time, she told me, "I'll leave a tincture for you in the mailbox. I'm gonna be leaving before you can come by, it'll be in the mailbox. You can pay me later." So, yeah, flexibility, with a kind of mutual trust. Like when I did that 20-minute treatment and was fishing for my check-book, and she said, "Next time." So, I feel like she goes out of her way, and I'm assuming I'm not completely unique in this. She's a teacher and a healer, and people whose vocation is healing, typically, unless you abuse the relationship, really try to help. Not all medical people are. I think some of the people are more research oriented. I feel that way about the genetic testing that I went through, that they were extremely caring and they broke bad news to me very well. They laid out my options in a way that I thought was very sensitive, but, they were also immediately asking me about whether I would be included in this study or that study, and I've never heard from them again.

The distinction the patient is making here between healing as a vocation, on the one hand, and being very competent and professional, on the other, is another common consideration for people who see CAM practitioners. The fact that acupuncture, Ayurvedic medicine, and chiropractic all have roots in spiritual traditions likely contributes to this sensitivity.

I: How would you recognize a healer?

R: That's a good question. It may be just a matter of a kind of affinity because, I think, if I had wanted to pursue additional counseling with them, they would've probably been happy to see me again. It felt too clinical to me. And maybe it was because I walked in there, they performed a service, they knew they were gonna have bombshell information that would have repercussions for others in my family, and they helped me to think about how to tell and what to tell other people.

I think part of being a healer is maintaining that professional boundary where you don't pursue a patient, like if I don't call her, Mary doesn't call me, and say, "How come you haven't called?" I'm a client. So, it's not like a friendship in that sense. So I have to pursue the treatment. But if I do call, and it's been a couple of weeks or I've been traveling, she'll say, "Oh, how are you? I was thinking of you the other day." There's a relationship that I know is there. Of course, there's money that changes hands. But the money is, to me, a kind of an expression of the appreciation that she's helping me, and it's not like a fee for service. It's more like, "We have a relationship and I'm there when you need me, and it's up to you to decide when you need me, but I have your interest at heart." I'm not just a chart, you know?

So, I think there's a quality of presence it's hard to put my finger on. There's a concern that's also a warmth, I guess is the best way of putting it. There's a warmth that she has that my Zen teacher also has, that my therapist has, and I think if they didn't have that, I wouldn't have stuck with any of them, you know? Yeah, it's just a feeling that they really are listening. It's very deeply engaged, nonjudgmental listening that, that helps to make this a priority in my own life. You know, to listen to myself and to listen to other people.

And I go to them in part because it renews my own ability to listen to myself and to other people. So, it's almost like training, as well as treatment. You can tell she's really listening, and she'll bow her head for just a minute, and make a brief note, and then look up, and look at me again. So, I don't have the feeling it's a monologue. It's not like a lot of people that you talk to. It's just nervous energy where they're fussing with things, or they're rearranging things, or they've got a foot tapping or they're looking around. It's just this very still focusing. And it creates a kind of envelope in which it's okay to just be there and it has encouraged me to be also completely honest about what's going on. Sometimes it helps me to just sit there with her and try to figure out what's going on by talking to her.

The interview returns to this patient's experience with genetic testing.

I was 49 years old when this, my sister was 47 when she had her diagnosis, and they were extremely interested in every aspect of the family history of cancer suddenly, when this result came in. I actually am happy if my data helps other people. I was okay with that. I didn't feel exploited or anything. But they were not focused just on me and how to support me. Whereas, somebody like Mary, or my therapist, or even my Zen teacher. Of course, I'm part of a community there, so there's a whole context which our relationship also happens in, but when I meet with her one-on-one, face to face, it's just the two of us, and it's the same kind of space.

I think that what I've really valued about my relationship with Mary is—it's almost like this frequency she set up that I could get in tune with, helped me to, on some level, be willing, be open to exploring a different way of being, especially at this time in my life. And the cancer thing opened the door to that. It allowed me to say, "You know, the way you've been living, you can't live your whole life the way you were living when you were a graduate student. You're not a graduate student anymore." What I think I most value—there's actual healing, the treatments, and the support of my health, and attempts to get me back to health when I'm sick. But in particular the way she creates the space in which I felt like I could be open to a different way to be. I need the support that I don't fall back into my usual habits of body and mind. Staying up 'til all hours and then getting up at five o'clock in the morning to go sit, and drinking too much coffee, and not eating right, and ignoring that symptom that I know is gonna really come down like a ton of bricks if I don't pay attention to it. So it was an invitation that I felt like I could accept to acknowledge things that were presenting to me that I would otherwise probably have just pushed aside.

And Zen has worked in that same way. So they complement each other. It's a sort of synergy, that's part of why I keep going to Mary.

As is clear by the end of this interview, the practitioner this patient goes to is quite unusual. To begin with, she is functionally an "integrative health center" all by herself. In addition to acupuncture training, she is a nurse practitioner and is trained in traditional Appalachian herbal medicine. Equally remarkable is the attention she pays to her patient's work and life rhythms. There are also two very distinctive features of her sessions with this patient. The periods of significant silence the interviewee describes are a major departure from conventional medical practices. Silence is nowhere a part of conventional biomedicine. Health care focused on maintaining balance and finding a still point is something new. Related to the presence of comfortable silences is the fact that sessions with this clinician are also of "unpredictable length." This flexibility allows her to move with the patient's needs on a given day and to respond to unexpected developments. Freedom like this is made possible for many CAM practitioners in part by the fact that many of them are not enmeshed in insurance or reimbursement systems. In some cases, this is because of insurance company policies. In others, it is the choice of the clinician who prefers to work with patients as they see fit. This choice is itself made possible because most CAM practices are low-tech operations that require minimal capital. Nonetheless, all of this is consistent with an ethics of health care that more and more people are finding satisfying and fulfilling.

Unsurprisingly, people who put a high priority on relationships and who are proactive about sustaining their health tend to seek out CAM practitioners, a wide variety of whom are available in today's healthcare marketplace. As this instructive and candid interview makes evident, what distinguishes "complementary and alternative medicine" goes far beyond a laundry list of unfamiliar but effective treatments and colorful terminologies. These practices, if extended far enough, could provide an entirely different approach to health and wholeness.

"WE ALL WANT THE SAME THINGS"

That dying can be a healing process is a very old theme, but one made problematic for a culture in which death, as the British historian Arnold Toynbee said, is "un-American."[8] In one sense we all know we are going to die, since our species has been doing it for so long. Yet philosophers from Socrates to the present have insisted, as Montaigne put it, that "to philosophize is to learn to die" and that authentic life is always a "being toward death," suggesting that whatever dying is about, it is not easily approached.[9] Efforts to postpone the moment of death by both patients and their grieving families is a common occurrence in major medical centers, where there is an extensive range of options for aggressive treatment and life support. Avoidance of death and the desire to prolong our life as long as possible are habits of mind and heart deeply embedded in our culture. Such behaviors may be rooted in the evolution of human adaptive strategies and linked in some way to our survival. But the maladaptive human and financial costs of contemporary forms of death avoidance are considerable.[10]

Contemporary discussions of death range from the religious to the psychological to the medical. Many religious traditions have clear beliefs and teachings about life beyond death: reincarnation, an afterlife, the survival of one's descendants, and spiritual reincorporation into some larger whole. Psychiatrist Kübler-Ross has offered assurances of the possibilities of personal growth in her discussion of five common stances people take when confronting their own death: denial, anger, bargaining, depression, and acceptance.[11] And more recently, the rapid development of palliative care as a medical subspecialty and the increasing use of hospice care at the end of life provide assurances about alleviating two of the most prominent fears about dying—that we will die in unrelieved pain, and that we will die alone, in an alien setting.

Largely absent from contemporary interpretations is any detailed description of the daily life of the dying person in hospice care. Likewise missing is any detailed exploration of the mundane ways in which dying can be a healing process.[12] In the interview that follows, this patient testifies to what she sees and feels and knows about how her life has changed since her terminal diagnosis. Some of these changes have to do with the nitty-gritty of living while dying. Others have to do with the many kinds and levels of healing she experienced. The events and turns in her story are not uncommon, but her insights about these common experiences are sharp, trenchant, and embody wisdom about things seldom discussed.

The interview took place in the patient's home. The text presented here is less than half the total transcript of an interview that lasted just short of two hours. The length of the interview is noteworthy. When the interview began the patient was confined to her couch, unable to answer her doorbell, and wondering aloud whether she should have agreed to the visit because of her pain. In the midst of the interview, the patient began readjusting her position—sitting up, removing pillows, leaning across the coffee table. At the end of the conversation she walked the interviewer to the door.

I: What we're trying to do is learn things that will help improve care for patients and we can't do it without people like you helping us out.

R: Well the question I wanted answered the most, nobody would answer for me and that was, how long do I have to live? I had one doctor who told me in May that I had six months to a year to live. This was May of last year. So I'm way past the six months and now I'm past the year mark.

I: Did they talk to you about why they don't answer that question?

R: They just said there's no way they can tell. I think closer to the end it's easier for them, because I had an appointment to meet with Dr. O who is my GI specialist.

I: So you talked to her about this question?

R: And she says that she has no way of telling me, but we knew from the beginning that I was terminal, so the idea was to keep the quality of life as good as possible as long as possible. And the way Dr. O worked was that I was on several different chemotherapies. I would be on one until it obviously had stopped working. So then I would go on another one and then with the help of things like MRIs, other scans, she could tell how effective the drugs were. And when one stopped being effective then she would put me on another one and she put me on one that was so expensive, like $5,000 for a little bottle of pills. I've actually had two like that...what in the world was it called? And oftentimes she would change the dosage on them.

I had an appointment to see her two weeks from this past Monday, but she called me and asked me to come in if I could. And I have a very good friend that I have taken with me to all of my doctor appointments, this is one of the things I would just recommend so much to anyone going for any kind of treatment, that you have an advocate with you at all times. You need two sets of ears listening and they're gonna be different interpretations of what was said, and someone to just help remember with you what was said.

That went well with Dr. O from the beginning, but she got irritated with me. You know in the beginning it was, "Oh please Dr. O I want to be here for my daughter's birthday," which was in October. "I wanna be here for Thanksgiving. I wanna be here for Christmas," I mean it just went on and on.

I: She was frustrated with that?

R: No, what frustrated her was me asking her to give me some estimate of how long I thought I had to live. Until you reach a stage...she realized looking at my lab tests and also the growth from manually feeling where the tumor was, that the tumor was just growing away and she called me and told me to quit taking everything that I was taking.

Note here the complexity of truth-telling for a hospice doctor and the dying patient's hunger for truth. There are so many factors at play—medical, psychological, and spiritual. More than most other clinicians, those working with dying patients are pressured to prognosticate. The honesty, the effort, and the courage required on both sides are enormous.

R: She called me and wanted me to come in. When I did, she told me, she said, "I was not sure if you would still be alive to keep this appointment." And then I tried to pin her down. But you know I figured in her mind there is no further treatment, and so I might as well get my body off the poison it has been on for so long.

The course of the illness, it's not gone the way anybody ever told me it would go. This business with the lymphedema, it's been one of the most painful things I've been through and there is no pain medication that will work short of Dilaudid, which will make me sleep all of the time, and once I get on it, for all intents and purposes, that's when my life ends. You know I want to be able to communicate very well with other people. I don't want to be just one more piece of meat that's going through the butcher shop that day. And I have felt that way on quite a few occasions.

I: Can you describe what the person is doing when you feel like you're a piece of meat in the butcher shop?

R: Yeah, well it's not really what they're doing, it's what they're not doing. I'm just the next person on the assembly line.

I: So it's important for you to behave in such a way that doesn't disrupt the assembly line?

R: Absolutely and when I have, it's not been pretty. One of the worst departments over there [in the cancer center] is the radiology and oncology... where they actually treat you with radiation. I got a doctor who was running late. He found out when he came in to see me that he actually had another patient ahead of me and that just really set him off and so when he came in he wasn't even gonna sit down. He stood there and he turned and I hadn't had a chance to ask him a single question, and as he started out the door, "Anything else?" And I said, "Yes," and he comes back in, "I have quite a few questions." He started out the door again, "Anything else?" Well, as he started out the door the third time, I broke into tears and I said, "Yes there's a lot else that I need to know, but you obviously are too busy to stop and take time with me." At which point he did come in and sit down. I'll give him that.

And the people in that department are the very same way. I did not come across a single one that I would describe as compassionate or truly interested. Here's the problem they had with me that day. I have lost all of my body fat on the upper part of my body and that includes my back, which it's just like knobs all the way down. So when I got in the room where they were going to set me up for the future treatments, they wanted me to lie on a plastic table with nothing underneath me. I'd had radiation treatments before and I knew it didn't have to be that way. And I said, "I'm sorry I can't do this, I'm too uncomfortable." So they said, "Well you know you have to" and I said, "No I don't, I can get up and leave. I don't have to do anything." Well that really set them off.

And so the next thing that appeared was the little foam pad about this thick to go on the table. Well then I told them that I couldn't lie with my head back like this, I've got a metal rod in my neck, plus I have cancer in my spine now. Well I'd have to. No I don't have to. Well the next thing I know they come out with a thing that is something for someone to put their head in. They've got them, but it makes their job more difficult because they have to redo the measurements, the measurements they take for the radiation are based on someone lying on that bare table. So they have to go in and change those measurements and then they have to each time they set up. And not only that, when I'm lying I have to have something under my knees.

And the last thing, which is really awful, is I have arthritis and cancer in the bones in my shoulders, so they wanted me to lie like this with my arms back flat and once again, I can't do that. Well you have to do it, well I can't and I don't have to. I mean this was the way the visit went. So sure enough these things appeared that would hold my arms up. So as I got ready to leave that day and they just didn't like it at all and I didn't feel well you know, I was in a lot of pain as it was, and before I left, I said, "Ladies I want you to remember that behind every face that comes in this door is a human being that is suffering, or they wouldn't be here." "Oh, we love our patients" and then this one lady pip-squeak who looked like she was about 20 years old, said, "I know what you're going through, my father had the same thing." And I said, "Have you had it?" It's that kind of attitude.

Treatments that exacerbate pain are particularly problematic when death is imminent—especially when much of the pain could so easily be avoided. The treatment the patient describes—aimed at palliative care—turns out to be excruciating in and of itself. To some degree, this insensitivity to dying patients is a side effect of our overall focus on "curing" and "preventing dying." It also has to do, of course, with efforts to cut costs and streamline medical systems. But here we get a stark look at the daily cost in the lives of patients.

R: Whereas in the treatment room the attitude is different, but the treatment room is aggravating too because you don't have any privacy. They've got chairs crammed in there and they're asking you about your bowel movements and everything else with all these people sitting around and then they even at times have to expose you so they stand a nurse with a sheet on either side you know. They just have outgrown the space they have and I say, when you outgrow the space you stop accepting patients, you know, don't punish them.

And then there was one time in the treatment room when they actually lied to me about something, they made a mistake. And they didn't want Dr. O to find out about it. She's very strict. She runs a tight ship. I went in there and I waited and I waited and I waited. Normally I go get my meds, my labs done, and they're able to read those labs instantaneously. And what they were checking for, the reason I had to do the labs, was to make sure that my white blood count was not too low...that was the main reason to check that out and so my appointment was at 9:00 and the nurse that I had been assigned to that day didn't come in until 9:45, but they didn't bother to tell me that. They just let me sit. And then they said, they hadn't gotten my labs back and that's why I'd been waiting. And I said to this nurse, "I didn't just fall off the turnip truck. If you will look at this lab sheet it will tell you what time it was completed and when it was sent to you."

Well, she started crying because she was the one who had told me all of these things that weren't true. She didn't bother to tell me that there was no one there to give me the chemo. She didn't tell me the truth; they were trying to put it off on someone else because they didn't want Dr. O to know they had screwed up so badly. I even asked to see Dr. O, not about this, I had a question for her. Normally you talk with one of her nurses and then they go back to her, which was fine with me. But she was not there that day and that was the other thing: when my lab report came back, my white blood count and the other measure that she used, they were low...and so they didn't know whether or not to give me chemo. And the other doctor on her team was not there either.

I: So there was nobody to cover, no physician.

R: Nobody. And so because of that, they weren't going to give me the chemo. I said, "If you will pull my past labs out, you will find that every time it's above 3.0 she has given me chemo on those days." They hadn't bothered to look at that, they were trying to make a decision on their own without looking back at the records to see what had been done in the past.

I: Can you describe one of the better experiences?

R: Well a good experience would be when your buzzer goes off within a reasonable amount of time. That's the first part of a good experience—not having to wait too long. And then when someone comes and gets you with a smile on their face and they know who you are, they remember your name. And then they want to make sure that you're comfortable, do you need a pillow? Do you need a blanket? And they just don't need to act harried around their patients. If they are, they should keep it to themselves because that energy translates and transfers right into the patient.

And then there are the ones who chat you up about this and that and the other and you share a laugh with them...not everybody can work in that department. You know it's a very hard place to work physically because you're on your feet so much. You have your patients, but you are also expected to help out other patients. If a buzzer goes off for someone that isn't your patient and it's time to switch the drugs, you're supposed to jump on board and help out. But, they have lots of wonderful, wonderful nurses that are concerned if you're being treated with dignity and compassion and to make it as pain-free as possible.

I was there a lot more than I would've liked to have been there. Because of the fact that I was getting an infusion also, which is not chemo, but it was a drug to strengthen my bones...so I had to go in for that also. I saw a lot of them. And there were many, many that I had just wonderful fun relationships with, who were always glad to see me and I was always glad to see them. I'm sure coming across as a cruel task master, but consider the amount of money that they get paid for the treatment.

This is another thing. They need to respect your modesty, which they don't. They're just so used to seeing half naked people or they don't always think about the fact that you don't like lying up there nude from the waist up with other people coming in and out of the room.

Being a patient is very often simply humiliating, even in the best of circumstances. But the patient is here talking about how much of what used to be considered "common decency" has been dropped in medical contexts, typically in the name of efficiency and economy. The testimony of the dying brings this tendency to demean the person into sharp relief.

I: As you think back through any of the physicians that you've seen, are there things that stand out as positive experiences, about the way they established relationships, maybe in the first couple of visits? How would you describe those?

R: In the radiation department the second time I went, I saw a different doctor and he was totally opposite. He was great, you know. He answered questions without my even having to ask 'em. He sat down and he wanted to know how the entire experience was going for me. And I had a bad sunburn on the inside of my esophagus, because I was having radiation treatments up here. Well, this doctor actually sat down and wrote out a prescription for me and said, here this will help you eat and drink, without my having to say, "Don't you have something you can give me for this?"

One of the very worst experiences . . . I had a procedure called chemoembolization. It's where they go in your femoral artery just like they do for a stent in your heart, only they're directing that catheter directly to your liver to shoot the chemo. I had asked the doctor what the side effects would be, and he said that I'd feel like I had the flu. I asked for how long and he said about four weeks. When he said the flu, if he had said bubonic plague it would've been more accurate. I have never been so sick, I lost 30 pounds in this one month's time. I had ulcers all in my mouth and all the way down my esophagus.

He never one time—he took off and went to Europe—had set up an appointment for me to go back and just look at things like my labs. Well I ended up in the hospital, I could hardly walk I was so weak and called Dr. O and begged for an appointment. They told me to come on in. I had no white blood cells practically and I was anemic. I had to have two units of blood and then I had this problem with my throat. None of which, well my [hospice] nurse told me that it was like thrush, and that there was treatment for it. So I called over and talked with this doctor's nurse and said, "They've told me at the hospice there's a treatment for this, that this is thrush," and she said, "I'll have to ask him." So she calls me back and she says, "He gives you the procedure, he doesn't know how to treat thrush." So when I went to Dr. O, it made her angry and she said, "Yeah they do the procedure and then they turn you over to someone else to mop up after them." Well when I went back for my last appointment, I had a very

young doctor—my other doctor was in Europe—and I told
him about this whole experience and he said, "We do order
blood tests on our patients. We order one once a week."

As the interview progresses the picture of a patient surrounded by
highly specialized medical teams gradually gives way to images of
this patient in community with her friends and her family.

R: I have a very good friend who has helped me in the doctors'
offices. She goes with me to all the doctor's appointments
that I have. And I have another friend who does all of my
financial stuff. She did my tax returns for '08 and '09. So she's
familiar anyway because I'll have one more tax return and
that will be an estate tax return and we're already working on
that, getting organized so that you know it won't be a lot for
her to do.

I: Well you're blessed to have these two friends, it's an extraordinary gift.

R: There is no blessing like it. I've had friends who came out of
the woodwork, friends I hadn't seen in a long time or who
I only saw infrequently. I have been treated so lovingly, it's
just been overwhelming to me. I'm so very grateful that I had
this year to spend this time with these people. It's interesting.
The two friends who have helped me the most have both said
to me that they consider it a privilege to be able to do this.
Which goes to show that many times the people in your life
are willing to do more to help you out than one might have
guessed. So we just need to ask.

What's the most anybody can say? They can say no. And
then you're no different in the way you were before you asked.
But I have found that my faith has strengthened my friend-
ships and my relationships with my children. You know it's
been amazing to me.

We've all faced this with the idea that I was going to get
through this the best way I possibly could and continue to try

to do things for other people as long as I could. Taking my energy and using it like that has also given this year a lot of quality. I'm not afraid of dying. The one thing that I am afraid of is suffering, which I am suffering right now and they told me at hospice that I would not suffer. But they do not have an effective pain medication for this business with my legs.

The patient's descriptions of her "healing relationships" continue to turn to her more intimate acquaintances and her family. Watching this "inward" progression from healthcare professionals, to friends, to family allows us to see the various kinds of healing—ranging from pain relief to spiritual reconciliation—that can take place in the process of dying.

R: I've got a daughter who lives over in the next county and she has two girls, my grandchildren are 10 and 12, and I have found explaining this process to them has been helpful to me in understanding it.

I: How has it helped? Because explaining it to them has got to be different from explaining to your friends or even your daughters.

R: Well, I'll tell you how I told them and then I think you'll understand that as I told them this, it gave me more clarity myself. So they were over here, they've known all along that I was ill, but they did not know how ill and I think they just kinda figured out that I was dying, but no one had ever told them that. So they were over here visiting with me and they had been outside. I don't know what the acorns are like where you live, but we just have a plethora of acorns and they cover the ground in the spring and in the beds you've got all these little oak trees coming up. Well I don't know how two kids have gotten through school to be 10 and 12 years old and did not know that an oak tree, that it comes from an acorn. They did not know that. I was taking them downtown to a show at the theater and when we finished, we came back here to the house and I thought, this has been a really good day and I need to talk to them a little bit more. So we went and got something to drink and we sat out here on the deck and I said, "Girls, Nana wants to talk to you about something. You know that acorn that we looked at; I want you to tell me what you think the life cycle of this acorn would be."

And we talked about how the acorn sprouted its little roots and its top, and it began growing and that if it grew long enough it would be as big as these other trees, but that took a long time. I was asking them questions to get these responses back from them and then we talked about what the oak tree did during its lifetime, how it started out tiny, how it grew to be large, how it provided shade and oxygen and the things that it did that were good during its life.

I said, "This tree is probably a couple hundred years old. What do you think happens to the tree eventually?" And they were sitting there not saying much of anything and then Alice said, "It dies." And I said, "Yes." and I said, "Our lives are just like that. We start out just like the acorn, we start out as just tiny little things and if we are nurtured we grow." And I said, "Nana has been through that stage where I was the big oak tree, and in the process of that, I have done things, I've had a wonderful life." I told them how just one of the best things that had ever happened to me was their being born, but I said, "Nana is at the end of this time though, and the illness I have is going to cause me to die at some point in the fairly near future."

I could tell they were really mulling this over and I told them they could ask me any questions they wanted to ask me, that I didn't mind answering questions, that I wasn't afraid. I assured them of that and I talked to them a little bit about my view of death and what I thought would happen to me. As I said, my own faith has been strengthened, not faith as far as a denomination or a religion, but my belief in God is stronger than it ever was.

But what I have found is that there are not enough people who recognize that we all want the same things, you know we really do all want the same things out of life. And that we really need to help each other to get them.

There are a lot of things I still don't have any answers to and that was another thing the girls and I had a chance to talk about was how, what happens to us after we're gone is probably so amazing that our brain doesn't even have words, that we don't have words to describe it.

I: People tend to try to protect children from the dying. But mostly it seems they're protecting themselves, because the children generally know what's going on. What children really need is just the kind of conversation that you had with these girls. And children are often better able to carry on conversations about death than adults, which sounds like that's what you found.

R: I think it's because they're closer to having been where I'm going. But they wouldn't understand that if I told them that way.

I: No they wouldn't. I may get this wrong, but I think it's Wordsworth who said that we come from that place "trailing clouds of glory." And that one thing that happens unfortunately—the clouds are still there—but we just lose touch with that place.

As the interview neared its end, the patient returned to the printed copy of the interview guide that she held.

R1: Okay. Let's see here [looking at the interview guide questions], what would you say that your providers have done during the time you have been seeing them that has most helped you deal with your illness? I thought that was such a good question. It's being honest with me and not acting as though this isn't happening. People need to have some understanding of what's wrong with them. What can and can't be done. This is maybe a lot to ask of a doctor or of the other people that work with the doctor, but I don't think it is. I think that's part of their job is to tell you what's wrong, what can happen, and what they can do about it. It's the most important thing and then recognizing that it is happening and that what's happening is something special.

We completed 14 interviews for this project with patients who were enrolled in hospice programs. There was a poignancy to each of these conversations. In part because the interview itself was the first and the last time we would be talking with each patient. The bald fact of their upcoming death was ever-present. But there was added poignancy in the fact that none of these patients would live to see what we made of their contributions, or to see how what they offered affected the students we asked them to imagine addressing and advising. Many of the 14 patients we interviewed displayed an honesty and depth that was evident to us during the interviews and even more so as we prepared their transcripts. As T. S. Eliot puts it in his *Four Quartets*: "the communication of the dead is tongued with fire beyond the language of the living."[13]

We close with a more complete quotation from Wordsworth's "Ode: Intimations of Immortality from Recollections of Early Childhood," which was alluded to in the course of the interview.[14] The passage serves to frame both experiences of hope and healing, while offering rich context for appreciating our last patient's insights into the origins and destinies of human beings.

> Our birth is but a sleep and a forgetting:
> The Soul that rises with us, our life's Star,
> Hath had elsewhere its setting,
> And cometh from afar:
> Not in entire forgetfulness,
> And not in utter nakedness,
> But trailing clouds of glory do we come
> From God, who is our home:
> Heaven lies about us in our infancy!

What is special about these journeys is precisely that they show us with clarity and insight the larger world we inhabit when we are patients. They reveal to us the selves hidden or latent beyond every one of us when we are conventionally labeled as "patients." We see relationships deepen as their "carrying capacity" increases. We see how crises develop and how they are held and resolved. These are not people made over into some idealized version of our humanity, whether as autonomous agent or consumer or good or bad patient. There is a sense in which we know, from conducting these interviews, what they are like as people. And this is the point. By virtue of their generosity, we get an intimate look at the subtle nuances of patient vulnerability and the contours of professional responsiveness. Ethics is the effort to discern what is valuable about the human shape of things, seeing deeper into the values that each of us carries, beyond the commercial and professional renderings. This is what is on display, quite vividly, in these three journeys.

[5]

BEING A PATIENT

The Moral Field

Throughout this volume we have argued that being a patient is a unique moral experience, with its own structure, rhythm, and horizon. In this chapter we turn explicitly to the moral domain. What we propose is an account of moral life rooted in vulnerability and responsiveness, indeed, just the kind of vulnerability and responsiveness that is patently on display in the interactions between patients and their clinicians in the previous chapters. This is the moral life that sooner or later we all recognize: a life anchored in the body and in time, sprung of relationships, inherently social, inextricably natural, and inevitably moral.

The distinctive structure, rhythm, and horizon of being a patient can be summarized as follows. The *structure* is dictated by the patient's vulnerability and results in what we call *doubled-agency*. Doubled-agency is meant to suggest additional strength or power, as when pieces of cloth are folded or "doubled" to make a stronger seam. There is likewise the suggestion of two actors, retaining separate identities, working toward a common goal, for example, doubles in tennis, double-teaming in basketball, or a double-play in baseball. Likewise it includes the sense of doubling our effort or our redoubled efforts.

The *rhythm* is one of mutual responsiveness—this responsiveness is an interactive dance between patient and clinician. There are of course short dances and long ones, but there is always this rhythm of reciprocity and teamwork in successful clinical encounters and in ongoing therapeutic relationships.

The *horizon* in view is always healing, however tacit; curing or fixing is usually also in view, but not always. By contrast, a hope for healing is never out of view. The inevitability of death is also always present, if most often unspoken. This structure, rhythm, and horizon provide the shape and the contour for the patient's moral agency, and the clinician's as well.

Examining a rudimentary case will be helpful here. We begin with a practitioner describing for us a satisfying simple examination, diagnosis, prognosis, and treatment:

> I saw a case of Erythrasma the other day. Erythrasma is an infection caused by *Corynebacterium*, and it's a skin infection and it has a very characteristic glow, a coral red glow when you shine a Woods lamp on it; and so this patient came in who was not having any real results in getting rid of his rash. I shined the light on it and it fluoresced floral; and the treatment with erythromycin is going to [make him] a happy guy because no one has helped him before.[1]

What we see displayed here in its most elementary form is the structure of doubled-agency as it operates in the patient-world. The skin's vulnerability, its ongoing instability and its constant interaction at the boundary of our bodies, is a condition ripe for disorders. In this case, the patient had a simple rash. But any rash, as patients and dermatologists readily testify, stands immediately as an appeal for help—to the patient and the patient's family and friends. The patient shows the arm, offers the appeal to the clinician, who, in turn, responds. The patient accepts the diagnosis and prescription, and applies the medication. The patient's skin becomes healthy again, which allows him to move back into the full range of potential his life and world offer him.

The structures and rhythms of doubled-agency are evident at every level of clinical interaction, from the simplest to the most complex. We can watch as they play out through the particular idioms and constructs and the habits and habitations of the medical world that the patient moves into by seeking help.

PHENOMENOLOGY OF BEING A PATIENT

Bringing in a practitioner makes two people active in a patient's health.[2] But bringing in a practitioner is not just a doubling of agency; it also entails at least a partial subordination of the patient's agency to the clinician's. This complex form of agency entails an extra layer of risk for the patient. But it also involves extra power—and it is the deployment of this latter in service of the health of the patient that justifies the voluntary subordination to the clinician and its attendant risks.

Agency—Clinician and Patient

Doubled-Capacity

The most prominent feature, then, of being a patient is the change in who is "in charge" in our lives. There is a change in agency; the practitioner becomes our agent, acting on our behalf and in our place, in certain prescribed areas related to health and illness.[3] We subordinate ourselves to our practitioner; we subject ourselves to examinations and to treatments. The relationship of clinician and patient is thus, as enacted and as realized, an intentionally asymmetrical one. We move into this distinctive type of relationship trusting that our practitioners will handle their agency in our lives well, with responsibility and with care.

We take a risk in giving over such power to another. But we take this risk because additional power, an added capacity, is just what we need or want in our lives at those moments. Because our own agency is compromised, we are willing to give over our power to another. We cannot evaluate our situation or fully understand what is going on in our lives; we cannot extricate ourselves from the predicament.

Often, part of the reason that we cannot extricate ourselves is that we have, in some measure, turned against ourselves. One piece is grating (perhaps literally) on another. One sector is at war with another. Our bodies have literally turned against us. We need a clinician because we cannot recover our unity or balance without outside assistance. We need someone to augment our agency. The detailed analyses in this chapter are more systematic explications of just what this doubled-agency means, how it goes wrong, how it goes right, and the insights to be gleaned from it.

Doubled-Risk

There is a central paradox in deciding to become a patient—the paradox of adding risk to risk in order to get help. To whatever vulnerabilities, wounds, and disruptions are moving in our lives, we now add an additional risk: the possibility of a harmful even destructive experience with a practitioner.[4] We subjugate ourselves to this person, and they can then take advantage of our vulnerability and harm us or—far more often—are just not careful enough and we are harmed. But we take the risk because we figure the odds are better, even with the doubled-vulnerability, than we are going it on our own. We have already tried, in most cases, to go it on our own. We've consulted our local resources: our friends, our family, the Internet, the guy at work who says he's got the same problem, or a friend whose aunt is in the medical field.

We have given a taxonomy of how things go wrong in these relationships in chapter 3, but it is worth emphasizing a few of them to highlight our emphasis on risk.

1. There is the risk of not being seen or heard, of exposing your secrets, perhaps your guilt and shame, and finding yourself fundamentally ignored, as a person.
2. There is the risk of being judged for your condition, a condemnation of habits or lifestyle or perceived weaknesses.
3. There is the risk of having pain inflicted in examination and testing processes.
4. And there is the risk of harm being inflicted in the application, even the successful application, of requisite therapies.

Entering into the relationship with the clinician inevitably establishes a power differential—a differential that exists no matter how sensitive to this asymmetry a given clinician is. And, it should be noted, this doubling of the risk applies as well to the patient who is not ill, who is coming to a practitioner for a physical exam, or a "maintenance treatment." The differential, and the corresponding risk, are generally reduced the less vulnerable the patient is.

We want to take special care to emphasize that we are taking a far broader view of vulnerability than those definitions, institutional policies, and rules concerned with "at-risk" populations. These populations very often hold places in our society that put them at greater risk than the population at large. We intend here, however, to incorporate a range of examples and cases, of degrees and gradations, of subtle and gross discrepancies in power and vulnerability. Factors in the shifting currents of vulnerability and power include race, ethnicity, class, gender, education, state of health, and age. Other less often considered factors include nutrition, housing, clothing, job status, life stress, time of day, region of the country, neighborhood in the city, violence and trauma, and natural disaster. All of these elements— and an infinite many more—can be found at work in relationships and balances of agency and power between patients and clinicians.

The risk entailed in supplication, the surrender involved in accepting the authority of the clinician to greatly influence or even direct some aspects of our lives and to interact with our bodies in certain unusual and powerful ways, is at times a truly terrifying element of engaging with clinicians.

THE PATIENT-WORLD

Vulnerability and Responsiveness: The Moral Typography of the Patient

We will offer a picture of the moral life of patients that fits what we have learned, that emerges from the compelling features of our research findings, not one that is imported from the requirements of other disciplines, such as political philosophy, economics, or theology. Here, as always, the best direction is from the ground up, letting experiences show what theoretical framing and conceptual apparatus is needed, letting the experience drive the theory. Principle-based approaches in bioethics, largely derived from political philosophy, have long been criticized for their abstractness, their individualism, and their heavy emphasis on rationality.[5] Virtue-oriented approaches, often seen as the remedy to a principled approach, have enjoyed a recent resurgence, and in *Healers* we discussed some of the ways clinician healing skills could be recast as virtues.[6] But even virtues may not speak well and without modification to the patient's world and its particular moral dynamics. Medical ethics traditions are hardly more reliable guides for understanding the moral life of the patient, as we will argue in the next chapter. The clinician's world is not the patient's, and the differences should provide clues for how divergent from the medical model of moral agency a truly patient-centered ethics needs to be.

Within these contours, we argue that the key terms for moral analysis and understanding are *vulnerability* and *responsiveness*. The patient's body and self are intensely vulnerable. This requires an ethics that accentuates the responsive abilities of the clinician in recognizing, validating, and lessening the patient's vulnerability. It is fundamentally a matter of willingness to help the body while simultaneously holding the person intact. In extended relationships it means holding out reminders of the patient's more full self, or locating the full self in the new and more limited physical body, or helping the person adjust to a diminished, but still valuable, body and self. The patient's moral responsiveness means acknowledging the power of the clinician as healer, and finally enough agility of moral agency to refigure one's life values in light of a newly discovered and more fragile incarnation.

The patient's weakened agency leads to the need for an augmented power, so the ethical dimensions at this juncture center on the shape of this doubled-agency, which can be described as a partnership aimed at healing. A partnership not so aimed leads to exploitation and abuse.

At some point the patient's moral responsiveness must take the form of a willingness to take responsibility for healing, though this is not always simple or easy, either physically or morally. Clinicians must be willing to share the intent to heal and act on it—assuming authority and taking responsibility for its practice. This is the defining moral feature of clinical professionalism. There must be some degree of partnership. The quality of that partnership may well determine how far down the road of healing a patient travels. What is at stake is one's health and sometimes one's life itself. So in the everyday manifestations of the patient-clinician relationship, the quality of this partnership, because death is never too far from the horizon, involves an ethics of vulnerability and responsiveness and therefore an ethics of life and death.

It is worth noting that there are other specifics of enactment for other practices of doubled-agency. Doubled-agency is not only found in the world of patients and clinicians. Lawyers and clients are an example of another domain where this structure is readily apparent. Parents and children would be another. In every such "doubling," in each such partnering, we expect to find distinctive sets of subordinations of authority, responsibilities, and relinquishments. These specifics will, of course, differ from domain to domain. It is the distinctive sets of subordination having to do with clinicians and patients that is our focus here.

We would add, however, that the patient-field of doubled-agency is an especially promising one for gaining insight into an ethic of vulnerability and responsiveness. The distinctiveness of the patient version of doubled-agency is the urgency so often called for in treating the body's fundamental wounds. But it is this very distinctiveness that makes the more general features of doubled-agency stand out starkly and unmistakably. Once we have seen these features in the patient context, we can then look around and see that vulnerability and the appeal for partnership, for coupled- or joined-agency, is the rule in human life, and not the exception. It is in this sense that the vulnerability of illness is emblematic of human moral experience in its entirety.[7]

NUDGING HER ALONG

What does doubled-agency look like in action? How does it manifest itself in the dance of clinician and patient? In the following interview excerpts, a patient speaks of her primary care physician's way of "nudging" her along in three very different situations: her hip degeneration, her cancerous skin lesion, and her substance abuse. The patient's capacity as agent is compromised in very different ways in each of these situations, which makes her report especially instructive here.

> We have a chart that comes with us that they know which medications we're on and all this type of thing, but, he started pushing me about my hip, gently. It was worn out. Dr. K was very gentle. I was still getting the oxycodone but I had become so dependent on it. I did have a lot of pain... I was not ill. But anyway, he took care of my having my hip X-ray completed, made an appointment with the best orthopedic doctor in this town. I had no choice... and it's now four months since I've had my hip replaced. I've gotten along beautifully, beautifully.

The patient is having difficulty walking and is in significant pain. But she is also paralyzed, in terms of her own agency. She is unable to move forward or to move backward. And so together they take the first step of having the deteriorated hip replaced.

> Now the next nudging that he did, you could see this [pointing to moles on her arm] I wasn't paying a bit of attention to it, and he nudged me into having a biopsy... and it turned out that they were basal cell carcinoma, which I owe him candy now because I argued with him and I said they can't be. Well, he assured me they were. So, the biopsy came back positive, he was correct and he found me a good plastic surgeon, I have seen her... and I'm going to have these removed soon. Thanks to Dr. K, because I would've just let them sit there forever if he had not gently pushed me.... He does not say, do this or do that, ever. It's a matter of, "We need to check this out." "We need to think about this." Then you get, "We're gonna do it"—not dogmatically—but it's just a matter of very gently, "It's time for you to make up your mind."

This time there is a potential threat to the patient's life—basal cell carcinoma. But rather than being stuck, as before, this time the patient is in disagreement with her clinician. She resists his diagnosis of the lesion on her arm. The clinician continues "gently" to insist on it, but without commanding, without suggesting "noncompliant behavior." That is, he makes room for this woman he knows, while at the same time insisting that she act under his guidance to deal with the lesion.

We go back now to pain—and pain medication. Very tricky territory for a practitioner and a patient to negotiate together:

> I'm inclined to dig in my heels and chances are I didn't even listen as much as I should have. When I said Dr. K should've pushed, I should've listened, too. But I didn't deal with it; I dealt with it very poorly. And he had to confront that...and bless his heart that he did, that he put up with it, that's what I said, he should've pushed when I had dug in my heels. I had dug in my heels because I was stupid enough that I didn't realize how serious my condition had become.

The clinician is attuned, very finely attuned, to just how much "pushing" and "nudging" his patient would allow. But, more important, he was finely attuned to what degree of insistence on his part would avoid demeaning or humiliating his patient. That she might say later, "He should've pushed when I had dug in my heels," was likely made possible by the very fact that he did not push harder. A difficult passage was traversed, with the mutual relationship of respect and fondness still intact.

THE MORAL FIELD OF DOUBLED-AGENCY

In this section we give a more detailed exposition of the four basic structural components of the moral field of doubled-agency for patients that play themselves out in an ethic of vulnerability and

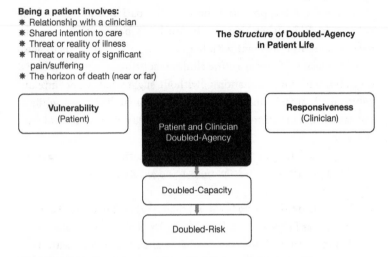

Being a patient involves:
* ✳ Relationship with a clinician
* ✳ Shared intention to care
* ✳ Threat or reality of illness
* ✳ Threat or reality of significant pain/suffering
* ✳ The horizon of death (near or far)

The *Structure* of Doubled-Agency in Patient Life

Vulnerability (Patient)

Patient and Clinician Doubled-Agency

Responsiveness (Clinician)

Doubled-Capacity

Doubled-Risk

DIAGRAM 5.1 The *Structure* of Doubled-Agency in Patient Life

response. In the next section we will provide examples from our interviews that ground these reflections (see diagram 5.1).

The Body as Vulnerable

In the patient-world we find ourselves compromised and at odds with aspects of our world and within ourselves—and at risk or vulnerable at our core because of that. [8] At risk because we ourselves are fluid, complex, and uncoordinated in our multiplicities that we can hardly even claim to have a single self, except when the body is threatened. But even then, there is no simple, singular identity—indeed, *no single* bodily experience. This multifaceted vulnerability renders solo agency impossible and suggests in retrospect that fundamentally, despite our fantasies of independence, it never existed. We are always coupled to some degree. Our essential social interdependence, though often forgotten, is as clear as our need for food, shelter, and warmth; as clear as our hunger for the nurture and love of our families; as clear as the necessity for networks of extended family and friendship throughout our lives. And these are *all* needs that are sharply accentuated with advanced age.

Serious illness is a stark reminder of our deep interdependence— a reminder of the special coupling with clinicians that our immediate physical dis-ability, and the specter of continuing vulnerability, make necessary. Sometimes this vulnerability presents suddenly; sometimes it grows over several years.

The Body as Appeal

The body makes an ethical claim simply by standing before us. That appeal, written as it is into our very physical natures, becomes more urgent as our bodies become less upright, in times of pain, disability, and dying.[9] The person is, in a very precise sense, always a supplicant self. When we become a patient, we offer the body as appeal in a very particular way, and to very particular people. A patient's body presents as vulnerable, whether in illness or in health, and with or without speech. This is no less true when we are hauled unconscious into the emergency department or when we present for our annual checkup. There are also those common instances when our presentation of vulnerability is unintended or unconscious. For example, we arrive in our clinician's office for a routine visit, and she notices a change in our gait or a shift in our bearing that begs for examination. The body is the primordial expression of appeal, even when fully upright, since we are never free from risk, always vulnerable, never free of our basic needs for others, never without interdependence. This is the case even when we are well and our vulnerability is out of our focal awareness.

Response of the Other

The body presents itself, ill or healthy, and in so doing *is* an appeal. The healing practitioner is one who accepts the authority of that appeal, and responds to it. Conversely, clinicians who refuse the authority of the appeal of the patient's body are unlikely to establish healing relationships with patients. Unfortunately, in our present medical system, this is a phenomenon we as patients encounter all too often.

The supplicant appeal of the body opens avenues for response. The clinician comes forward to establish a relationship, with the intent to help and with the willingness to take responsibility and assume authority. The patient in turn seeks partnership and, as we have emphasized, is always making unequal alliances in terms of power and risk. What each person in that partnership understands by that coupled-agency is critical: it can either diminish or increase vulnerability. How those partnerships are formed, why they work initially, and how they are sustained over time—can be of major importance in our lives.

Acknowledgment of the Other

We become patients by acknowledging a clinician's responses to us, by displaying a readiness and a willingness to participate in a coordinated movement toward healing. But this conferring of authority on the clinician by the patient is born out of trust, as well as out of need. One must trust the "office," the socially legitimated role, to which one subjugates oneself—in this case, the office of "healthcare practitioner." But one has also to trust the particular individual officially "certified" to fill that office—in this case, a practitioner with a name and a face.

The patient steps forward into this unique relationship and in so doing accepts the clinician's authority, hoping for help in the face of illness, suffering, and ultimately, death. This means that in choosing to be a patient, one is deliberately taking a subjugated position in the hope of achieving a goal one cannot reach alone. This is the paradox we spoke of earlier; by relinquishing one kind of power, the patient gains access to another.

THE RHYTHM OF DOUBLED-AGENCY IN PATIENT LIFE

Frighteningly enough, this body of ours, this body that is the core and the pulse of our world, goes through regular cycles and rhythms

of uncertainty and incapacity. There is no such thing as health without illness or illness without health. Moving with these rhythms, we
go through periods of time when we are not patients, and periods of
time when we are. When we are patients we get examined, probed,
and questioned. We get diagnosed, we receive prognoses, and we
undergo treatments. We all realize, as well, that there are degrees of
being a patient; there are times when we are more deeply enmeshed
in the medical world than others.

To grasp more fully these degrees and rhythms, we need to
delineate more precisely the salient features of the doubled-agency
in patient life. The body that undergoes medical examination may
be described as "the body in limbo." The past we thought we understood—the body we have relied on—is now altered. There is now
uncertainty about its meaning and status. With uncertainty in the
present and the past, the future is now clouded.

- The process of being diagnosed and receiving a prognosis is
  experienced as an exploration of the past as it manifests in
  the present (diagnosis) and an exploration of the future as it
  is implicit in the present (prognosis).
- The treatments we undergo as patients are encompassed in
  our efforts as persons to realize our full potential and possibilities. What was uncertain when the body was in limbo
  now shows itself in reorientation—whether that is a course
  we consider healing or a course we consider a continuation of
  an illness. Either way, the ambiguity is, for now, resolved.

Becoming a patient, however, does not at all confine one to a passive
role. The patient has activities one undertakes to fill the role of patient,
for example, following a medication regimen, doing physical therapy,
keeping tracking of blood sugars. The patient is also an active partner with the clinician in many other activities. One collaborates with
the cardiologist as a heart catheterization is in process, one reports
on pain and other bodily sensations while physicals are being done,
one works with a practitioner to develop a comprehensive history,

and one prepares for and does the rehab after a major surgery. When we speak here of "doubled-agency," we are speaking of *two agents at work*, together pursuing a shared goal.[10]

It must be noted, however, that keeping one's own agency intact and engaged when one is a patient takes constant effort and sometimes incredible determination. At times this means reclaiming one's agency from one's illness or injury. At other times, it means continuing to maintain oneself as a person even while subordinated to and in the grip of the medical world.

It is, in turn, important to see that in any given situation of doubled-agency *both* parties—the one "taking on responsibility" and the one "under the care of"—stand to benefit if the goal is attained, though in very different ways. And likewise, both are at risk, though again in very different ways, if the goal is not attained. Typically, of course, the risk is greater for the one "under the care of." Which is why we always emphasize the trust involved on the patient's part, and the responsibility on the clinician's.

Let's take a moment now to review our analytical approach. First we find "the body in limbo," poised amid several possible paths, courses of action, and events. Next, we experience an inability to move out of that place on one's own toward the realization of some portion of the body's potentialities for wholeness. We hope to come out of that limbo state able to actualize and reclaim some portion of the possibilities our lives offer us. It is the movement through limbo, through a full assessment of past and future in the present and then on to healing that we observe as the rhythms of doubled-agency unfold (see diagram 5.2).

KEEPING TIME, HOLDING THE BODY

Careful study of the experience of patients, we are arguing, calls attention to an ethic of vulnerability and responsiveness. That same careful study also makes it clear that the patient's experience is governed by the rhythms of illness. Illness courses through time. Illness—and

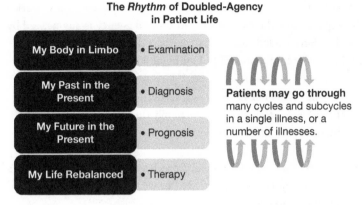

DIAGRAM 5.2 The *Rhythm* of Doubled-Agency in Patient Life

health—is, in fact, a way of naming how the body moves through time. The patient is never static, nor is the body. A diagnosis is a diagnosis of the course of one's lifetime, as well as of one's body. The same holds for prognosis. An examination of the body occurs in time and alters time; so too does a treatment. A medical intervention is an intervention in time as much as in body. The patient is vulnerable in body and time—never one without the other. In this exact sense, *we are beings of time, more than beings in time*. More precisely, we are not fixed and isolated entities inserted into moving time. We are essentially time ourselves, just as we *are* motion, from cellular structures on up to the biographical and on out into the communal.

We want now to take two more complex excerpts from our interviews and explore how the dynamics of vulnerability and responsiveness come into play when we become patients. We will also be looking to see how co-operative accomplishments of the doubled-agent, of the partnership of patient with clinician, manifest in situations where the weight of time is so confounding.

The first example has to do with shared agency focused on treatment with very explicit goals in view. It involves, for example, speech therapists working with the patient quoted in chapter 1 who had a climbing accident deep in the Canadian wilderness that resulted in major brain damage and a subsequent series of surgeries. Notice throughout how the patient's compromised agency is augmented by the clinicians' skilled agency in such a way that healing took place. We begin with a blunt statement of vulnerability and appeal.

> The speech therapists were wonderful. I mean, I didn't have a choice 'cause I was driven by my family three times a week to see these people and I was still kind of brain scrambled.

The therapy that follows is a very precise response to the patient's very specific injury. This specificity lies within the larger dynamic of appeal and response.

> But it was literally like, "Put the red box on the red box." They had this computer thing they would have me do and it's put the red box on the red polygon and the yellow star on the yellow star, and I would use the mouse and click and drag and then next visit they'd be like, "Okay well let's see if you can do that one faster."

Taking responsibility in the doubling of agency means responding as precisely as possible to the impairment at hand and offering the patient genuine possibilities for recovery, for further realization of his body. A body that, in this case, is decidedly in limbo in the critical area of speech and language.

> I: So they're trying to get the wires back and the speech ...
>
> R: Yeah. And once I started to get through that then it was things like reading different little logic puzzles and trying to figure those out and then I was doing lots of Sudoku.
>
> I: So what were they like during this process?
>
> R: Those people would take their time out to stay.... When I had gotten into tears over am I ever gonna be normal again, and them taking the time to talk. And I just remember the real kindness of those people, and then the kindness of the physical therapists. 'Cause I couldn't even move my left arm.

> Now it's perfect but at first I was just like retarded mentally
> and had practically no use of my left arm.

Seldom is there only one area of vulnerability. Here we have emotional vulnerability, motor limitations, and cognitive impairments. The skilled clinician moves among these levels and balances what is needed to acknowledge and respond to each, at the right time and in the most appropriate way.

> And the patience that they used and the encouragement and the
> relaxed kind of attitude that they had. "Hey, you're not gonna get
> better today and that's okay. But you will. It's not gonna happen
> overnight, but hey, give yourself a break. This is gonna take some
> time. No big deal. We're gonna work with you." The patience
> really felt good.

What we don't see but can extrapolate is a long history of exams, many surgeries and setbacks, leaps forward and steady growth. What remains constant is the patient's ongoing vulnerability and the appeal he makes that his clinicians continue to respond to—from the emergency response teams to the brain surgeons to the speech therapists. The patient's body remains in limbo throughout, with more uncertainty in some areas than in others. More promise of recovery and full realization in some areas than in others. And the patient, as part of the shared quest for healing, continues to seek and receive the clinician's response—and to assent to the treatment, the regime, and the authority carried for him by his clinicians.

Our next account illustrates the kind of diagnosis and entailed prognosis that, in the moment they occur, change *everything*. What was hidden in the past is made known in the present; what is hidden and often feared in the future becomes clear in the present. This may be a simple change, it may be complex, it may be monumental. In the exam the clinician's eye becomes touch, in the diagnosis the clinician's word becomes touch. That touch may be gentle and, as in this case, it may be too sharp.

Prior to the diagnosis and the prognosis, there is a period where the body is in limbo. For this hospice patient, a startling life event— "an aneurysm in my right aorta and it blew out." After the initial lifesaving work had been done, there followed a not unfamiliar confusion about the proper diagnosis of an underlying condition. Then finally comes the all-too-decisive diagnosis, and the total reshaping of his life and the sharp clarity of end-of-life issues.

> I: Could you tell me a little bit about what it was, what it was like when you first enrolled [in hospice]?
>
> R: Well, I'll back up a step; I'll not drag it out. On October the 12th I had an aneurysm in my right aorta and it blew out, I bled. And the doctor said I was one of the very few that lived and tell about it. Most times you drop, but I came through it and he told me it would take at least six months for me to get my strength back. I didn't have any strength at all. So I went to work hard on it…. But my strength wasn't picking back up like I thought it should. And so I went to the VA Hospital just to see if I could get some tests run and those people down there were great. They started running tests.

Our own time threatens to become governed by diagnosis and prognosis, where the past is judged, no *livable* present exists, and the future is prejudged. One has, in effect, in this zone, no time of one's own— it is subsumed into the medical world.

> And he couldn't find anything wrong except he did tell me I was 63 years old. I wasn't 18 anymore, takes a little longer than six months. But he says, "Let's go back to where the problem started with your aneurysm." And so he did a CAT scan on it and when the scan brushed my lower lung and he said, "I see something there that I don't like."

The depth of the vulnerability of the patient's body is slow to reveal itself. There are small cycles of appeal, response, and acknowledgment as the patient journeys through more examinations and diagnoses. As long as this man remains a patient, the shape of medical time remains an overlay, an often oppressive overlay, on his living time—and here, in turn, his dying time. Notice below how the patient reasserts his own sense of his own life's time against the imperatives of the clinic.

And so they did an ultrasound and then he came back and did a whole CAT scan. It did show up in my lung and a spot on my liver and here and there. And he said, "Well, a lot of times it'll try to go to your head, too. Let's check that." So they did an MRI and it showed that I had a tumor in my head.... And that doctor said, "Just to be sure, I want to send you to [the regional medical center] and let them look at all this." So she put it on a DVD for me and I carried it over there the next morning. They wanted to go in and remove that tumor. They said they wouldn't get all the tissues, so I'd still have to have radiation and chemo.

Notice how the ongoing *acquiescence* of the patient to his clinicians is brought to an end by the patient himself.

I felt like they was a little pushy over there, maybe they wasn't, but you dropped a bomb on me. I said I've got to pray about this and think about it. "Oh, no, we've got to get you scheduled." I said, "No." So we left. And we were supposed to have been back at 3:00. My daughter said, "What do you want to do?" I said, "I'm going home."

Paradoxically, it is the accurate diagnosis that gives this patient the power to extricate himself from the pathology-focused medical system and to recover much of the agency he had given over during the examination period. His prognosis—terminal as it was—set him free to make the last movements of his life in the way most meaningful to him. Acknowledgment of the authority of the medical world ended as the patient began his final moves of gracious *acquiescence* to the larger rhythms of living and the horizon of death.

It is into our longing and fear, into our remembrance and anticipation, that we invite our clinicians, hoping for them to tip the balances toward life, toward fulfillment, toward healing. In so doing, we are enjoined to confront the uncertainties of our lives. And enjoined, even driven, to do so in ways that expose our vulnerabilities with special emphasis and urgency.

[6]

RETHINKING
HEALTHCARE ETHICS
The Patient's Moral Authority

The health of our bodies is the fundamental pulse of our life-world and determines our capacity for access to that world in all its manifestations. When our bodies are compromised, as they inevitably will be, we seek assistance. And to get this assistance, we offer and then submit ourselves to the care of practitioners, always with the tacit agreement that they are willing and able to help us. This is what we have learned from listening to the patients we interviewed. How this goes; how vulnerability is recognized and responded to; how the partnerships of doubled-agency are framed, sustained, and interpreted are the core patient experiences that must inform healthcare ethics.

As we better understand the moral field of being a patient it becomes readily apparent that contemporary approaches of both bioethics and medical ethics have severe limitations. Each speaks to formal obligations and professional standards rather than patient experiences. Each is centered on the agency of the clinician rather than the frame of the patient, and both speak in an idiom that is largely foreign to patients' lives. Working out of our patient interview transcripts we argue that a more grounded ethics is needed, one that is truly serious about being patient-centered.[1] We call this new ethics for patient care simply "healthcare ethics," to differentiate it both from bioethics and from professional codes of ethics devised by doctors and other clinicians. By this term we avoid naming a given profession, such as medical ethics or nursing ethics. We want to indicate that this is an ethic that should occupy center stage for anyone who aims to offer help to patients, whatever their training. We advocate that this be the everyday core ethic for not only physicians and nurses, but also respiratory therapists, medical social workers, hospital chaplains—essentially anyone working professionally in health care, including consulting bioethicists. It should be noted that we are confronted with a new and complementary patient authority, with patients naming and shaping the moral scene and by doing so providing a clear corrective to professionals and ethicists who have been the dominant players in framing the moral agenda. In framing an ethics that is truly appropriate to health care, and not borrowed or adapted from another realm of human activity, we are offering a different method for moral reflection, one that begins with the embodied patient and builds out. This is the moral dimension of healing interactions and "patient-centered" care. The patient's moral authority is finally not just the authority to refuse care or the right to be treated with respect and dignity. The real authority of patients is having their framework of experience taken seriously as a basic normative structure for shaping the moral imagination of those who are committed to helping them heal.

THE REMOTENESS OF BIOETHICS PRINCIPLES

The three principles that have dominated bioethical discussion for decades—respect for autonomy, beneficence, and justice[2]—all presuppose, in their most common renderings, an Enlightenment view of moral agents as solo, largely unencumbered actors. This view of agency represents a philosophical response to political circumstances that occurred during the Enlightenment period.[3] It answers the question of why governments should confer liberties or rights to individuals by constructing an ideal self-determining citizen. Most of us admit as a matter of course that, on a daily basis, no moral agent ever realizes this ideal. Yet we continue to use it as guide for our reflection, our decision making, and our policy. When, however, we look at the patient's world we see that not only is this ideal impossible to meet, but that ongoing efforts to meet these requirements tend to take us in the wrong direction. Continuing to use these concepts as core elements of ethical analysis and as basic tools to gauge the adequacy of clinical decisions leads us away from the heart of the routine moral activity between clinicians and patients.[4] In the long run an exclusively principle-oriented bioethics runs the risk of becoming irrelevant, because it misunderstands the patients' fundamental vulnerability, which constitutes their moral authority.

In their efforts to operationalize the insights of the European Enlightenment, bioethicists have worked, almost since the inception of the field, with a principle-centered ethics, circling around the familiar triumvirate, with nonmaleficence now often included as a refinement. Yet again and again the same fundamental problem arises with this principle-based approach. These concepts may be argued for (cogently, if not persuasively) as abstract frameworks. But when we seek to apply them to areas of clinical life and patient experience, they often seem formal and clumsy, tailored for issues that are not routinely encountered. One reason is that the phenomena of clinical interactions are of such complexity and richness that using these or any principles as the chief mode of understanding morality undervalues this richness. If these principles are imposed on circumstances for which they were not designed, they can easily do violence to the intricate fabric of moral life—somewhat akin to using an axe to operate when what is needed is a scalpel. Our problem with this set of three or four principles is not that they are useless, but that they often fail to address the structure and rhythms of routine health care. In this sense they may function well for "big decisions" and policy ethics, but they are often not suitable for daily use.

We will discuss briefly the four chief principles of bioethics and assess each in light of our doubled-agency model:

Respect for Autonomy. The description of the patient's moral field that we have developed suggests that the usefulness of the concept of autonomy is actually quite limited. Typically, autonomy is essential for clarifying the ethical situation at the point where a patient arrives at a major decision. But it is not at all helpful in clarifying the dynamics of how a person—a vulnerable, wounded person—*becomes* a patient and relates more routinely to the clinician. The appeal of the patient and the response of the practitioner occur almost instantaneously. A person clearly does decide, most of the time, to become a patient of a particular clinician, but the sense of self as an autonomous agent is typically not in the foreground. Given that, and the urgency and uncertainty often involved, the conditions typically associated with respecting a patient's autonomy obscure the patient's need for a partner. The patient looks for trust, confidence, and assurances of safety when working with a clinician.

What most patients want is to be an active member in making decisions about their care; they want what we have described above as doubled-agency. In that partnership, they count on clear professional recommendations. Our experience as clinical ethics consultants has taught us that respecting the patient's autonomy is too often taken by clinicians as a license to evade the burden of the decision—together with responsibility for its outcomes—and pass it to the patient or the patient's family. This is sometimes expressed as follows: "Here are your options, now you have to choose."[5] The key ethical element in many of these situations is not the danger of trampling on the autonomy of patients or their surrogates, but a question of the degree of trust and confidence between the healthcare team and the family or the patient. It is worth emphasizing that patients and families seldom arrive in clinics and hospitals with strong capacities for autonomous choice. Such choosing is only possible for anyone, and especially in health care, in a context of enablement, when choosing is actively supported by an environment of trust, solid information, and recommendations that appreciate that patients are also persons with lives outside the immediate context of care. The presence of community is, after all, an essential precondition for the emergence of any form of autonomous activity.

If respect for autonomy provides minimal guidance during the inception and development of the clinician-patient relationship and through key decision-points along the way, then at what point is this principle helpful? We find that an approach that emphasizes respect for patient autonomy has a larger and more proximate place in areas such as the dissolution of a relationship. If the doubled-agency partnership is strained or breaks down, there may be a distinct juncture at which the patient's needs must claim the right to shift from doubled-agency back to single-agency. This movement is a movement rooted in a lack of recognition of or respect for patient autonomy. Autonomy at this moment means essentially having the option of saying "no" or of insisting on negotiating where and when the patient will or will not acquiesce. The concept of autonomy can help clarify the dynamics of this shift from doubled-agency to single-agency. It can remind us, for example, that no one is authorized to treat another without consent. But even here autonomy is of little help in understanding why the breakdown occurs, why the trust essential to doubled-agency has disappeared. It appears only as a final arbiter, as a trump card against paternalism.

Beneficence. This ancient principle is likewise of limited usefulness. As with autonomy, it shows its relevance most clearly in situations when the doubled-agency of patient and practitioner is in jeopardy, but has not yet reached the point of dissolution. Patients of course seek help from clinicians only because benevolence, or good intention, is assumed. When the confidence and trust the patient has in the goodwill of the clinician begins to be strained, there are often efforts to clarify the goals of the partnership. At this juncture a patient might be asking, "Are my assumptions about the clinician's benevolence reflected in beneficent actions and attitudes?" "Is my well-being still the primary focus in this partnership?" This juncture requires renewed emphasis on the patient's healing as the primary intent of that partnership. Beneficence has as its goal the patient's good, and healing is understood as one aspect of the broader goal of beneficence.[6] But as long as the doubled-agency functions well in its concrete pursuit of the patient's good, the principle of beneficence remains in the background. Beneficence becomes a focal point *only* when it comes into doubt. More precise analysis of healing and the intent to heal can typically be provided by studying how the medical frame alters the patient's life and life prospects, and how clinician and patient work together within that frame toward healing. For example, when patients and practitioners deliberate in earnest about treatment options they are not concerned with beneficence but rather the more specific question of benefit: "Which therapy will make my life better?" Except when their partnership is in question, analysis of the structure and rhythms of relationships clarifies the moral lives of patients and practitioners in more precise and exacting ways than the principle of beneficence.

Nonmaleficence. This principle is treated by some bioethicists as being distinct from beneficence. The obligation to avoid doing harm and actively prevent harm is thought by some to be the oldest and most stringent duty of physicians. It is expressed in the Hippocratic tradition as *primum non nocere* (first, or above all, do no harm). It can be viewed as a counterpart to beneficence in its assumptive presence in healthcare encounters, without which there would be little reason for patients to seek help from clinicians. Its importance should never be minimized, given that so many diagnostic and therapeutic maneuvers—as well as all prescription drugs—can have damaging effects. Still, we contend that as important as this principle is as a premise for a clinical exchange, and as an ongoing boundary marker in qualifying the effects of beneficent intentions, it is not a focal point of the routine dynamic of clinician-patient interactions. It comes into play in a critical way as a clinician tries to sort out how a relationship could be compromised or damaged, such as with a breach of confidentiality, or when specific remedies have unintentional harmful side effects. Then, of course, a harm/benefit calculus is clearly in order, and a principle underlining the obligation to refrain from harm or minimize it is a salutary reminder. This use of nonmaleficence might arise often in some invasive specialties, or in cancer care, and clearly in the care of the severely and terminally ill. But even there it gives only rough or approximate guidance for negotiating complex territory. The nuance of the harm/benefit calculus is always mediated through a relationship or set of relationships. Nonmaleficence is at best a marker of the costs and limits of intervention. Generally, it is too generic a norm to provide guidance in discerning how harm might be done in the routine fluctuations of clinician-patient relationships.

Justice. The utility of the concept of justice, unlike that of autonomy, beneficence, and nonmaleficence, most often comes to the fore not when doubled-agency is strained or breaking down, but before it gets started. A person is wounded; the body makes its appeal. And then there is no response. Becoming a patient proves difficult. Usually this absence of response, this difficulty, is a matter of access to clinicians. This lack of access typically centers on failures of institutional structures, financial incentives, or sometimes geography. Justice will in such cases be an absolutely central consideration in addressing the policy and economics of healthcare resources. For example, there may be no response to the patient's appeal because a clinician, often functioning under efficiency and profitability mandates, refuses access to care. This is usually not an individual decision, but a result of policies put in place by a group practice or a larger institution to meet goals of profitability. Here we face injustice of another kind. Injustices can also occur on the individual level when specific refusals of access are related to race or to insurance or socioeconomic status. Such cases raise fundamental questions of equality and justice. But once the doubled-agency of clinician and patient is established, justice is usually too abstract and generic a term to be applied with the precision required to be helpful.

If we turn to a more pedestrian and functional notion of justice, such as "fairness," there is arguably more traction for discussing the interactions of clinicians and patients. A simple example: a patient feels she is being treated unfairly because there was no time to ask questions in an appointment. We can also imagine more troubling situations, such as when advocacy for a patient is curtailed because the care required becomes financially unprofitable, when the patient requires additional time for reassurance or explanation about a diagnosis, or when a patient is simply abandoned as uninteresting or undeserving or too difficult. In all but the more extreme instances, it is not possible to be clear about the meaning of fairness without understanding the particularized history of the doubled-agency at work, and knowing the rhythms of vulnerability and responsiveness that have marked such relationships prior to the point of strain or dissolution.

Notably, however, fairness as construed in this primary healthcare context does not involve seeking balances of benefits and burdens in relationships of reciprocity between autonomous agents. Fairness here is about recognizing and respecting the roles and responsibilities the partners in doubled-agency carry as they come together with the intent of healing the patient. Fairness in this sense always has multiple dimensions. Patients may treat clinicians unfairly, they may violate the trust of that relationship by using the clinician to access controlled substances or by refusing to follow the guidance of the clinicians on matters essential to the patient's healing. In turn, clinicians may treat patients unfairly and may violate their trust by engaging them primarily as consumers and fee-units, or by ignoring patient concerns and questions. Yet even here the dynamics of doubled-agency—with the power discrepancies, the subtle agreements, and the fluctuating obligations they all always involve—offer a finer-grained analysis than can the notion of fairness alone.

We are arguing that the four principles—respect for autonomy, beneficence, nonmaleficence, and justice—are not focal points of the usual relationship dynamics between patients and clinicians. We are claiming that the four principles are typically called into play at the assumptive level (beneficence and nonmaleficence) or when the more fundamental structures of healing interactions are poorly established, are breached, or are otherwise called into question (autonomy and justice). To clarify: We are making a very specific criticism here of the principle-oriented approach to bioethics and medical ethics. We are not saying that principles are completely unserviceable for guiding ethical reflection and practice, nor are we saying that they have no place in the overall moral sensibility of healthcare professionals. We clearly need principles, and we clearly need the four principles we have discussed. For example, respect for patient autonomy can figure prominently in the overall aims of a healthcare practice and in the design of healthcare incentive plans. Some managed care plans and patient compliance structures seem to disregard patient autonomy; they also tend to disregard beneficence as an expression of the judgment of practitioners for what constitutes best care. Likewise, a healthcare system that does not seek justice in universal access would be morally bankrupt.

As useful as these and other principles are, they do not speak effectively or convincingly to the most basic moral aspects of clinician-patient interaction. They leave open the question of how ethically complex relationships in clinical settings ought to be understood. This is what our patient informants have shown us, and what we seek here to emphasize and explore. Any professional ethics that ignores the dynamic of vulnerability and the responsiveness that gives form and structure to healing interactions will be overlooking something rudimentary and essential.

Consider the following two situations.

1. *"Do I keep going back?"* You become a patient because your body is vulnerable. This sets in motion the sequence of appeal to the clinician, the response of the clinician, and then the patient's acceptance of doubled-agency. Suppose now that you are enrolled as someone's patient and you have been seeing this practitioner for three or four months. Gradually you come to feel you aren't being treated well. Perhaps your treatments are not helpful, or you don't get adequate explanations. Perhaps you feel you are being ignored, or maybe you are given someone else's test results by mistake. How are you to think this through? Add to that the potential that your practitioner may start to think of you as a "noncompliant patient," one of her "difficult patients."

The standard response to such a scenario for those schooled in bioethics would be to urge you to think in terms of your rights as a patient and focus on considering yourself an autonomous agent.

But you are a patient only when you are in a relationship with a clinician. You are a patient, that is, only because you have accepted, however provisionally, that you are not an independently functioning, autonomous agent. In a doubled-agency partnership there are sets of ongoing negotiations, which notions of independence and autonomy typically obscure. In addition, assertions of autonomy can lead to seeking a kind of freedom that is rarely possible, usually not desirable, and occasionally harmful. Attempting to establish oneself as the isolated, unilateral decision maker may well mark the end of the power and protection afforded by doubled-agency with a clinician. When this crisis occurs it is often unclear to patients whether they can find another practitioner who will provide the needed help when it is needed.

On the other hand, there are situations in which you may want to leave a clinician who is providing appropriate care, but you don't want to hear what she has to say. Exploring whether you might be wrong about the proper direction of your care is one of the benefits of effective doubled-agency. But an overemphasis on protecting your autonomy might incline you to dissolve the partnership because of unwanted advice, not of bad advice.

But suppose, after all is said and done, it becomes clear that you are finally ready to end the partnership with your practitioner, reclaim your complete autonomy, and say, "no more." Even so, you remain vulnerable and in need of help. You may be autonomous in choosing a new medical partner, but autonomy as a stand-alone guide does not resolve your ongoing vulnerability and can render this central facet of your situation invisible.

In sum: A model of autonomy is usually helpful only at certain well-defined and infrequent points in a relationship, and when used in more routine situations of health care it can actually be counterproductive. The model can easily mislead patients and clinicians alike about the nature of their relationship. Beneficence and nonmaleficence are important, we have argued, but are routinely out of focus and are much too general to be of use in understanding the daily back-and-forth dynamics of working with clinicians. Justice is of limited usefulness *within* a relationship, and its range of application is more often evident when no relationship is possible, or within a relationship when a basic clinical or patient norm has been breached.

2. *"How much truth do I tell?"* There are also situations of the opposite kind, where the question is not about the clinician's full engagement in the healing effort, but the patient's. Let us take the case of the patient who intentionally withholds from their practitioners information essential for his or her health care. We have in mind situations where a patient's distrust is operative at the beginning of the clinical relationship and is likely to be sustained the whole time the patient works with the clinician. Within our framework, we would discuss this in terms of partial acceptance. There can be, as we noted earlier, cycles of appeal and acquiescence between patient and clinician as their relationship matures. But here there is a refusal of adequate engagement by the patient that thwarts further development. Here we are looking at something more like this: "Yes, I will be your patient. But [the patient says to himself] I am not going to tell you about my substance abuse, about my sexual inclinations, about domestic violence." This degree of lack of trust—whether based on previous experience with clinicians and healthcare delivery systems or out of guilt, shame, or fear—prevents doubled-agency from its full potential. Savvy clinicians are alert to signs that this type of withholding and dissembling is taking place. There will be gaps in the evidence that make sense only if one accounts for substance abuse or violence in the home. But it takes a very skillful clinician and a courageous patient to overcome this kind of crippling dynamic.

When we look at what is involved when patients withhold information or lie and attempt to clarify the situation with the four principles, we find once more that they speak only to boundary conditions. They do not and cannot address the core structure and rhythms of a patient's engagement with a practitioner. Nor can they give guidance at the level of detail necessary to be truly helpful as patients and clinicians struggle toward maintaining healing relationships. For example, the easy read on withholding information from a clinician through the lens of autonomy is that it is the patient's right to do so, even when it jeopardizes care. Again, this is a "rights-trumping" mentality at work, rather than a more helpful emphasis on how trust and confidence can be developed and can function in the service of better care.[7]

Fortunately most clinicians are guided by their patients and constrained from too much ethical theorizing by the rhythms of daily practice that force them to deal with the subtlety of interpersonal exchange. Skilled clinicians learn from their patients how to see, how to act, and how to proceed at these levels. Bioethicists could also use such attentiveness to help adjust their concepts and methods into more serviceable tools.

Far from being inconsequential, it is the everyday detail and the most quotidian "decisions," with their cumulative effects, that frame the parameters of the big decisions patients are called on to make about their health care. Yet even this formulation assumes that we will all find ourselves faced with the classic dilemmas in bioethics, the ones highlighted in textbooks and much discussed in the media. But many, many patients make it through their lives without facing the dramatic issues that preoccupy bioethics. Our argument is that an ethics of vulnerability and responsiveness that attends carefully to the ebb and flow of the interactions between patients and clinicians can give access to the everyday ethics that matter most.[8]

THE NARCISSISM OF MEDICINE'S ETHICAL CODES

The title of this section may sound like a harsh judgment to many professionals, oriented as they claim to be to the well-being of their patients. Indeed, the preamble to the current American Medical

Association (AMA) Code of Medical Ethics states that it was developed "primarily for the benefit of the patient."[9] Despite this claim, it is medicine's view of the patient and medicine's benefit to the patient that shapes the code, such that narcissism is an apt description of the normative perspective the code reflects.

The narcissism we refer to here is not a psychiatric category, but a more general cultural category, here applied specifically to how health professions have conceived and articulated their basic moral commitments. In Greek mythology Narcissus was a beautiful youth who fell in love with his own reflected self-image. This excessive self-love was the result of a curse put on him when he refused the amorous advances of the goddess Echo. The consequence for Narcissus was a love that could never be fulfilled or consummated. Our contention is that professional codes of conduct and patient obligations have been defined since Hippocrates in terms that originate in the perceptions of the professionals themselves, with little or no influence from patients' understanding of what is at stake in the therapeutic encounter. The solo authoritative voice in these codes has been that of physicians. This does not mean such codes are useless or fundamentally wrong in their norms. There is much to admire in professional codes, and living up to their ideals has always been a worthy challenge. It does mean that the starting point and the articulation of these codes would differ dramatically had they been informed with the moral structure, rhythm, and horizon we have articulated in this volume.

More specifically, the Hippocratic oath was an admirable effort to identify those core features that would mark a profession that sought higher ideals than the medical tradesmen of ancient Greece.[10] It is also noteworthy that the oath was taken in secret and the teachings were by definition not to be disclosed to the uninitiated, including both patients and other practitioners. While the service obligations incurred by taking the oath are laudatory, their reference is exclusively to the physician's character, duties, and boundaries. The situation of the patient is not mentioned, except insofar as it indirectly shapes the occasion and context for the medical virtues. For example, entering a house "only for the good of my patients" and abstaining from sexual relations with anyone in the household is surely a good thing to aim for. But completely absent is the larger context of vulnerability and its presentation. Hence the narcissism involved in this ethic is its exclusive reference point to professional actions and attitudes. The narcissism is not in the idealism of the oath, but in the fact that the only agency in view is the physician's.

It would be tempting to think that in the modern era things improved and patients' perspectives were incorporated into medical ethics formulations. This has not occurred in any extant code of which we are aware. The sophistication of the contemporary codes and their accompanying principles are remarkable, and they clearly speak to the early twenty-first-century practitioner in ways that the Hippocratic oath cannot. Yet still one finds that each of the principles in the most recent version of the AMA code begins with the phrase "The physician shall ..."[11] To take another example, the excellent *Manual of the American College of Physicians*, which is routinely updated, speaks with candor about conflicts of interest and about the vigilance needed to place the patient's health above self-interest.[12] But these and other altruistic framings are presented as if they were completely the physician's invention and responsibility. Nowhere do they make reference to or seek guidance from patients' perceptions of what is wanted or needed for relationships to work therapeutically. Despite revisions, these core ingredients are still missing.

The reader might assume here that we are seeking to make yet another dint in professional sovereignty, in addition to those already made by consumerism and the increasing prominence of business norms and economic forces in health care. We have no such wish. Indeed, we believe that physician ethics has been substantially damaged by the compromises in professionalism that medicine has made over the past two decades. In this sense, the problems of professional ethics are problems of an overall anemic morality, marked by too little robustness of thought and action, and no real insulation from the hegemony of business values. If anything, physicians in particular have not pushed back hard enough, collectively and individually, against the dominance of the market. Medicine had its professional ethics compromised by business norms at least in part because it has been looking at its own reflection for so long, largely ignoring patients' perspectives. In brief, medicine has been confident about its own ability to identify the salient moral insights of patient care and articulate the norms that would govern actions and attitudes in that realm. The result is the absence of allies to help resist the commodification of its services. Medicine, in particular among the healthcare professions, has had to go it alone because morally it did not bring patients into the conversation and make common cause with them. The result is a diminution of medicine's moral authority, grounded in the vain presumption that only the professional can define what is morally important to the therapeutic relationship. Asking clinicians for less insular thinking in their ethical frameworks and urging them to listen carefully for what their patients need will allow them to reconsider the essentials of healthcare ethics. Including patients in the next formulation of their ethical principles would be an important step forward for medicine. An ethics for all healthcare professionals must be a joint project, a consummation of the key insights and phrasings of clinicians and patients in collaboration. Only if medicine can attend more carefully to the voices of patients and give those voices moral authority will it regain its moral footing.[13]

In this context, it is also important to discuss nursing and nursing ethics because of their central place in health care. Although nursing shares some of the same insular professional motifs of medicine, the tone and the principles in nursing codes show considerably more attention to the embodied values of the patient, and to the larger dynamics of healthcare interactions. For example, the code of the American Nursing Association (ANA) stresses the "dignity" of patients and is sensitive of the fact that people seeking care are compromised and vulnerable.[14] In addition, nursing formally endorses "compassion" as a central norm. The ANA code underlines this motif by discussing "the primacy of the patient's interest," and goes further by noting that patients are always in a "network of relationships" that informs and shapes their care.[15] Although the code does not say how one is to determine exactly what those patient interests are, there is at least a prominent place for patient voices in deciding what is important in health care. Perhaps the ANA code approaches patient relations so differently because nursing's origins were so directly shaped by human needs, suffering, and a service orientation. Or perhaps it is the more constant proximity to the patient, especially in hospital settings.[16] Whatever the reasons, we believe that nursing succeeds in avoiding a simple mirroring of the ideals of its own self-image and provides an example for how a professional code can be congenial with what patients are saying about the ethics of health care.

MOVING FORWARD: OATHS AND EDUCATIONAL OPPORTUNITIES

The moral life . . . is something that goes on continually.

—Iris Murdoch

How should we move forward? We will offer recommendations of both a conceptual and pragmatic nature, and conclude with examples of how the vulnerability and responsiveness dynamic we have emphasized could be translated into a new ethics code for health care. We are also interested in new educational opportunities for learning the skills that lead to healthy therapeutic relationships. We hope others will take up this work where we leave off.

If the source for professional ethics that is absent or underrepresented in current codal formulations is the patient's perspective, healthcare leaders would do well to invite a range of articulate and thoughtful patients into the conversation. Form focus groups and talk at length with individual patients, not with the idea of accommodating or "satisfying" them, which would be patronizing, but with an agenda of respectful attention to learn how to speak to the core elements of the relationship within professional codes. What we have presented here is just the beginning, and there is much to learn from an extended dialogue. There is no reason to think that doctors or other healthcare professionals are better than patients at discerning these core elements. Hearing patients talk about healing requires a rare but important assumption: that we can learn about differences while refraining from hierarchical judgments. Patient perspectives will be different from those of professionals, and diverse among themselves, as our interviews have shown. But they are neither inferior nor superior morally. They are simply distinctive, and in their distinctiveness lies their value. They provide the antitoxin for professional temptations to moral chauvinism, and thus hold a unique authority in clinical interactions. If we really want to make health care patient-oriented, the first place to begin is with a better understanding of the moral orientations that patients bring. Patient-orientation should be understood not in terms of the idiosyncratic values each of us bring, still less in terms of some satisfaction or happiness index, but in terms of the structural needs and requirements for entering a healing relationship. In health care we know how to fix a great many things, but we are constantly learning and relearning how to heal.

Out of such an effort could come a jointly written and mutually supportable set of professional values, principles, and virtues, and a reciprocal set of patient values, principles, and virtues. One of the fortunate hallmarks of the late-twentieth-century and early-twenty-first-century healthcare ethics, at least at the local institutional level, is that there are now lists of patient responsibilities to complement lists of patient rights. To be sure, these lists reflect some of the same professional agenda-setting and lack of imagination that mark medical codes, precisely because they are often formulated and posted with little or no contribution from patients. They are doctors' and often hospitals' and healthcare systems' versions of what will make relationships work, and what will help institutions survive and flourish. For example, this agenda is evident in the obligation to show up on time for appointments, to pay one's medical and hospital bills, and to follow all hospital rules and regulations.[17] If a new twin set of moral understandings drawn from *both sides of the doubled-agency of care* were articulated, it could use the first person plural. It would be, between patients and clinicians, "our" code—not a doctor's code or an institutional list for patients of "their" obligations. Ownership is an essential aspect of the authority of any moral agreement and enhances the sense of obligation. Most Europeans speak about their national policies as "our" healthcare system, even when they are complaining. Americans can only talk about "the system," which means, of course, the system that is largely controlled and directed by the most powerful players, the citizen-patient not among them.

Revising the Medical Oath: A Beginning

Imagine a group of new doctors affirming an oath that included one or more of the following pledges.

- I will see my patients as equal to myself in value and dignity, whose injuries and anxieties have made them supplicants for care. Understanding and responding to them is what gives my work meaning and makes me a professional.
- I will always seek to identify the person behind and beyond the patient before me and his/her presenting symptoms.
- I understand healing as a gift that grows out of trusting and confident relationships, and I will work to develop the skills that nurture these relationships.
- I will strive to remember that the knowledge I hold can fix and sometimes cure, but that compassion is needed for true healing. In the work of healing, who I am is as important as what I know.
- I will find ways to nurture in myself those traits of heart and mind needed for my chosen profession. Among these are compassion, mindfulness, trustworthiness, courage and equanimity in the face of suffering, advocacy for my patients, and humility.

In offering these statements we are not, to be sure, suggesting a wholesale substitution for existing codes, just as we were not suggesting a complete dismantling of bioethics. For example, a medical code that did not have *primum non nocere*, or some similar injunction about the ever-present possibility of harming patients would be neither realistic nor morally honorable. But neither is a professional code that fails to incorporate patients' perspectives and that does not emphasize the need for compassion, the reality of patients' vulnerabilities, and the obligations to acquire relational skills and those traits of character that are most conducive to healing.

Educating Professionals Who Are Healers

We close this chapter with suggestions for the education of practitioners. These suggestions come from several sources. Clearly a new code of ethics is an impetus for rethinking educational priorities and learning strategies. Revising an ethics code is meaningful only if it is reflected in a revision in training priorities as well. An ethics code that does not reflect educational priorities would be a sham. A second impetus emerges as we locate the true sources of the patient's authority in the formation of doubled-agency. If the patient is neither a passive recipient of care as in the old paternalistic model, nor an independent negotiator in the newer autonomy model, but a partner in a relationship of doubled-agency, the teaching about how to form and sustain such joint-agency relationships must become a high priority. It is clear to anyone who has ever been a patient that we all have an enormous stake in how and what healthcare professionals are taught. This seems obvious, but it is often overlooked or deemphasized. After all, we put our lives into clinicians' hands with great regularity, so of course we have a stake not only in what they know, but in how well they can relate to us. Finally, we are prompted to reflect on the education of practitioners by the responses our patient interviewees gave to this question: "If you had a group of young clinicians before you now, what would you tell them was most important about how they treat their patients?" We have quoted some of their responses in other parts of the book. But their wisdom informs our thinking here in a particularly cogent way. Here are a few of the things they had to say:

"Tell those young people to remember that it's the patients who are living it."

"The doctor needs to do a good job—but so does the patient. It takes both."

"They've got to really care about their patients. Patients can always tell."

And simply, "Have good manners."

With these sources in mind we would emphasize two general educational guidelines:

1. Teach that relationships are the key to healing.[18]
2. Encourage medical students to get guidance from patients they meet while in training.

Below are questions we believe educators of healthcare professionals could ask:

1. Education begins with the attitudes, skills, and demeanors, the habits of mind and heart that students bring with them to their training. How can we better select students who can develop into healers, whose thoughts and actions will be truly patient-centered? Could patients be creatively incorporated into an admissions interview process, just as we now seek to integrate them effectively into every year of professional training?

2. What kinds of educational experiences are needed for students who as professionals will see patients every day they practice medicine who are in pain, anxious, ill, or injured? What attitudes and virtues must be cultivated for practitioners to survive and flourish under such conditions? What attitudes will be toxic for this activity, either for practitioners or patients or both?

3. How can we better teach students the interpersonal rewards of practicing medicine? How can we deflect the often overriding concern with material rewards that preoccupy students the nearer they move toward practicing on their own? While part of this problem is student debt, the tone, quality, and priorities of their educational experiences must also shape practice expectations for students.

4. How can professionals who excel in their responsiveness to patient vulnerability be better rewarded and supported? What can be done to sustain them as they exercise these essential skills? This is both an economic and a cultural question, not answerable by academic institutions alone. Still, academic institutions, as well as professional associations, could make leadership in this area a priority.

The quotation that opened this section is taken from Iris Murdoch's *The Sovereignty of Good*. Her book contains, among other things, a critique of the formal, Enlightenment tradition of ethics that dominated her education. A more extensive quote from Murdoch is a fitting epigram for our concluding section. "I can only choose within the world I can *see*," she says, "which implies that clear vision is a result of moral imagination and moral effort."[19] We have argued that the world of the patient can only be seen with the moral imagination and effort that comes from attending carefully to the vulnerability of the patient and the central role of clinician responsiveness. Murdoch also cites the critical role of attention, giving it a primary place in ethics: "We shall not be surprised that at crucial moments of choice most of the business of choosing is already over...[because] the exercise of our freedom is a small piecemeal business which goes on all the time and not a grandiose leaping about unimpeded at important moments."[20] It is in this sense that the moral life "goes on continually." The primary task of healthcare ethics, we would argue, would then be to learn to appreciate and navigate this continuous moral flow.

The rhythm of illness and health is finally not something unusual, unique, or special. It is simply part of the ongoing human flow of appeal and response. True, there are crises and traumas—the quagmires and enigmas of boundary cases at the edges of life and relationships. But these are always best engaged, when possible, against the background of everyday attention to health and illness, to the care of the body, and to the nurturing of life that animates all partnerships between patients and clinicians.

Much of the power of an ethics of vulnerability and response derives from its insistence that we recognize the many layers of vulnerability in our lives. Likewise, this approach turns our attention to the complexities of the back-and-forth between patients and clinicians in situations that can be fraught with peril and driven by urgency. Such recognition and attention gradually, perhaps inevitably, make room for an appreciation of the body in its finitude and in its mortality. Being a patient can teach us this; and a patient-centered ethics can teach us how to live fully and gracefully with this most fundamental truth.

Appendix

1. Research Design and Planning

What makes healthcare relationships therapeutic? Why do some interactions with clinicians succeed while others fail? Clinician responses to these questions were presented in *Healers: Extraordinary Clinicians at Work*, yet that study was confined to the professional interpretation of what is a complex and multifaceted dynamic. It was clear that a complementary study was needed, one that focused on patients' perspectives. Therefore, the research presented in this volume is intended as a complement to the earlier study.

A brief account of the evolution of the semistructured interview guide is illustrative of the overall design of the project. In the process of developing the interview guide, we started with prompts for patients to talk about their healthcare relationships and to reflect on factors, for example, clinician behaviors that contributed to the quality of these experiences. We expected that, like the clinicians, patients would be able to remember specific interactions that exhibited—or failed to exhibit—care and concern. Upon further reflection, convinced that the distinguishing features of healing interactions might emerge from the details of the patient's life, and not simply from clinical encounters per se, the scope of the instrument was expanded to give participants explicit prompts to discuss their relationships to their clinicians in reference to their larger life story. The structure of the interview guide was motivated by a general methodological commitment to let patients speak for themselves. How to achieve that goal became clearer during the analysis and writing stages. Healing relationships are best understood using multiple modes of analysis, including structured coding/modeling, phenomenological analysis, and narrative interpretation.

2. Data Collection: Semistructured Interviews

SAMPLING AND RECRUITMENT

Our recruitment strategy involved purposeful sampling. We invited a group of participants that likely had had at least one "good" relationship with a provider and that was sufficiently diverse to account for the differences in what it means to be a patient. We continued to invite participants until we reached saturation. We asked eight of the 50 practitioners from the previous study along with several practitioners not in the study to provide us with the names of four to five patients who might be interested in participating. These practitioners helped us recruit by identifying patients they believed had a significant story to tell about healing and the relational aspects of care. We provided letters to these practitioners, which they sent to selected patients, explaining the study, asking about their interest, and requesting permission to be contacted by a member of the research team. Fifty-eight participants gave us permission to talk with them and were enrolled in the study. Their demographic information is represented in the table below.

Table A.1 DEMOGRAPHICS OF PATIENTS INTERVIEWED

Gender

    Men   23

    Women   35

Race

    White/Caucasian   51

    Black/African American   7

Age

    20–39 7

    40–59 13

    60–69 12

    70–above 26

Education

    Some high school or completed high school   11

    Some college   7

    Completed college   20

    Master's/Doctoral   20

A central aim of the interview guide was to provide an opportunity for patients to tell the story of their relationship with one or more providers. Beginnings, critical junctures, and reflections over the course of relationships were of particular interest. We also wanted to provide patients an opportunity to reflect on why the relationship worked or did not work. What did they remember about their interactions? Could they recall specific behaviors that impressed or offended? These are the questions we asked:

1. How long have you had your current healthcare provider? How did you decide to make your first visit to him or her? What was going on in your life at that time?
2. Think back to your first visits with your provider. What did he or she do that made you want to keep coming back to him or her? How did you make that decision?
3. When you think about *your most recent visits* with your healthcare provider, can you remember some of the things he or she said or did that *showed care and concern*, or helped to build your relationship with them?
    - When you think of your *visits to any of your healthcare providers*, can you think of things that providers have said or done that *showed care and concern*, or helped to build the relationship?
4. Can you think of things your healthcare provider said or did *in these recent visits* that *failed to show care and concern*, or weakened your relationship with them?
    - When you think of your *visits to any of your healthcare providers*, can you think of things that providers have said or done that *failed to show care and concern*, or weakened the relationship?
5. Can you describe one or two of the most important moments or significant events that show what your relationship with your provider has been like?
6. What would you say that your provider has done during the time you have been seeing him or her that has most helped you deal with illness, or move toward healing?
7. How is your life different now than it was when _____ first became your healthcare provider?
8. Are there other things about patients' relationships with their healthcare providers that we have not asked about that you think we should consider in our study?

From November 2009 to August 2010, we conducted 55 interviews with a total of 58 participants. The research protocol as a whole and the interview guidelines were approved by the Institutional Review Board at Vanderbilt University Medical Center. All interviews were conducted by the authors in the southeastern United States. Interviews were face-to-face and were held at a time and place that was convenient for the patient. The conversations were audiotaped for accuracy. Compensation of $35 was offered to every participant. Most interviews lasted about an hour, but they ranged from 20 minutes to 2.5 hours.

3. Data Analysis

Theoretical models such as *holding clinical space* and *doubled-agency* were direct outcomes of our data analysis. Each of these models reflects a distinct mode of inquiry. Below is a brief description of how we arrived at these and similar constructs.

DEVELOPING A CODEBOOK

The authors of this book were the only ones involved in the coding process. We began by reading and rereading transcripts selected from over 1,600 transcript pages to gain a general familiarity with what participants were telling us. Next, three especially content-rich interviews were selected and coded by all three investigators. Each code name and its meaning were discussed, coding discrepancies were resolved, and consensus was established around a codebook. We then coded five additional transcripts to establish interrater reliability, and finally all transcripts were coded by at least two of us. The qualitative software, Atlas.ti, supported these efforts.

With three people coding, we had to determine very early in the process whether we were coding the material in roughly the same way. The need to establish reliability across coders promoted a habit of comparing, explaining, challenging, and revising coding decisions. This proved to be immensely helpful not only for determining criteria for coding but also for deepening our understanding of categories that tend to resist clear conceptual boundaries, for example, empathy or compassion. In grounded theory, this process is commonly referred to as *constant comparison*. Chapter 2, for example, benefited from this iterative process where models such as *holding clinical space* and *compassion* developed through comparison of numerous quotations across multiple codes.

One of the limitations of grounded theory as a strategy for qualitative analysis is that the coding process breaks up the narrative flow of the material. As we began coding, we decided to preserve vignettes and longer narratives because patients repeatedly expressed peak moments of their relationships with clinicians in these forms. Vignettes were compared and grouped by themes and many of these reinforced coded categories. For example, the vignette category "full presence" augmented the trait of "attentiveness." Other vignettes captured distinct relational outcomes such as "human bond." Longer narratives, such as "Ibuprofen and Love," in chapter 4 were selected because they are forceful illustrations of the full radiance of clinical relationships when they possess healing power. They also contained important themes related to specific healthcare domains, such as living with chronic disease and end-of-life care. These stories were edited to sharpen the focus on poignant descriptions of the interactions as they occurred in a larger biographical frame.

4. The Writing

The organization of the book reflects the multiple modes of analysis in our research process. Chapter 1 combines phenomenological analysis with narrative interpretation to present the experiential structures of being a patient. Chapters 2 and 3 utilize the structured coding and modeling to provide theoretical accounts of the factors that encourage and discourage healing relationships. In chapter 4, we emphasize the primary material and provide commentary sparingly. While we obtained a general consent for all our interviews, we returned for additional permission when using extensive verbatim quotes, specifically, from the two surviving interviewees described in chapter 4. In chapter 5, we returned to a phenomenological mode in setting out the moral field that defines what it means to be a patient. And finally chapter 6 argues for the implications of our findings on the field of bioethics.

We leave this project with deep gratitude for what we have learned, and a greater appreciation of the courage, resilience, and wisdom of the persons we interviewed.

NOTES

Introduction

1. David Schenck and Larry R. Churchill, *Healers: Extraordinary Clinicians at Work* (New York: Oxford University Press, 2012).
2. The three authors are listed alphabetically. Each of us contributed in substantial ways at every stage of the project, from writing the IRB proposal, doing the interviews, and coding the transcripts to finally drafting, editing, and rewriting the chapters.
3. We conducted 55 interviews, but the total number of patients interviewed was 58, since in a few instances we interviewed husband and wife together, both being cared for by the same clinician.

Chapter 1

1. Much has been written on the power of illness to transform our lives. Paradigmatic examples include Arthur W. Frank, *At the Will of the Body: Reflections on Illness* (Boston: Houghton Mifflin, 2002); Anatole Broyard, *Intoxicated by My Illness: And Other Writings on Life and Death*, comp. and ed. Alexandra Broyard (New York: Clarkson Potter, 1992); Reynolds Price, *A Whole New Life: An Illness and a Healing* (New York: Atheneum, 1994); Harold Brodkey, *This Wild Darkness: The Story of My Death* (New York: Holt, 1996); Audre Lorde, *The Cancer Journals*, special ed. (San Francisco: Aunt Lute Books, 1997); and Kay Redfield Jamison, *An Unquiet Mind: A Memoir of Moods and Madness* (New York: Vintage,

1996). For fuller treatment, see David Schenck and Larry R. Churchill, "Patient Perspectives: Healing from the Other Side of the Bed Rail," in *Healers: Extraordinary Clinicians at Work* (New York: Oxford University Press, 2012), pp. 129–68. We do not intend to duplicate that work here. What we want to do is look specifically at what it means to be a patient, whether one is ill or not.

2. Primary resources for further exploration of the themes of vulnerability, the body, and the life-world as we have developed them throughout this volume include Judith Butler, *Giving an Account of Oneself* (New York: Fordham University Press, 2005), and "Survivability, Vulnerability, Affect," in *Frames of War: When Is Life Grievable?* (New York: Verso, 2009), pp. 33–62; Emmanuel Levinas, *Totality and Infinity: An Essay on Exteriority*, trans. Alphonso Lingis (The Hague: Martinus Nijhoff, 1979), especially "Ethics and the Face," pp. 194–219; Erwin W. Straus, "The Upright Posture," *Psychiatric Quarterly* 26 (1952): 529–61; Maurice Merleau-Ponty, *The Visible and the Invisible*, ed. Claude Lefort, trans. Alphonso Lingis (Evanston: Northwestern University Press, 1968), especially "The Intertwining—The Chiasm," pp. 130–55. In addition, see Maurice Merleau-Ponty, *Phenomenology of Perception*, trans. Colin Smith (London: Routledge & Kegan Paul, 1962); Emmanuel Levinas, *Otherwise Than Being, or Beyond Essence*, trans. Alphonso Lingis (Pittsburgh, PA: Duquesne University Press, 1998), especially "Substitution," pp. 99–129; Helmuth Plessner, *Laughing and Crying: A Study of the Limits of Human Behavior*, trans. James Spencer Churchill and Marjorie Grene (Evanston: Northwestern University Press, 1970), and "On Human Expression," in *Phenomenology: Pure and Applied*, ed. Erwin W. Straus (Pittsburgh, PA: Duquesne University Press, 1964), pp. 63–74; Richard M. Zaner, *The Context of Self: A Phenomenological Inquiry Using Medicine as a Clue* (Athens: Ohio University Press, 1981); and David Schenck, "The Texture of Embodiment: Foundation for Medical Ethics," *Human Studies* 9, no. 1 (1986): 43–54.

3. We have stayed with the phrase "Deciding to Become a Patient" as the title for this section fully aware that being taken to the emergency department in a variety of acute conditions does not entail "deciding to become a patient." But the decision is made by someone, who acts as the surrogate decision maker. And when or if the patient returns to capacity, the patient decides whether or not to remain in "patient status."

4. We do not consider the material our interviewees shared with us to be "illness narratives," in the sense it is used by Arthur Kleinman, *The Illness Narratives: Suffering, Healing, and the Human Condition* (New York: Basic Books, 1988), or in a somewhat different sense by Rita Charon, *Narrative Medicine: Honoring the Stories of Illness* (New York: Oxford University

Press, 2006). What the interviews are fundamentally about is relationships between the patient and the clinician during health, illness, and recovery. Interchanges between interviewer and interviewee provided unique opportunities for exploring the deeper dynamics that allow healing relationships to be sustained and, in some paradigmatic cases, to flourish over an arc of decades.

Chapter 2

1. See the discussion of the "healthcare container" and "medical rites of passage" in David Schenck and Larry R. Churchill's *Healers: Extraordinary Clinicians at Work* (New York: Oxford University Press, 2012), pp. 26–47.
2. The importance of holding in both literal and symbolic senses is explored systematically in Donald W. Winnicott's *The Child, the Family, and the Outside World* (Harmondsworth, Middlesex, England: Penguin Books, 1964).
3. This finding mirrors the thinking of our expert clinicians as reported in Schenck and Churchill, *Healers*, pp. 6–8.
4. Kelli J. Swayden, Karen K. Anderson, Lynne M. Connelly, Jennifer S. Moran, Joan K. McMahon, and Paul M. Arnold, "Effect of Sitting vs. Standing on Perception of Provider Time at Bedside: A Pilot Study," *Patient Education and Counseling* 86 (February 2012): 166–71.
5. Medical resident at large university medical center, focus group interview by Joshua Perry, March 16, 2009, audio-recorded, Vanderbilt University, Nashville, TN.
6. Hippocrates, "On the Physician," cited in Ira M. Rutkow, *Surgery: An Illustrated History* (London: Mosby Elsevier Health Science, 1993), pp. 24–25 (emphasis added).
7. Jerome Groopman, *How Doctors Think* (Boston: Houghton Mifflin, 2007).
8. Francis W. Peabody, "The Care of the Patient," *JAMA* 88, no. 12 (1927): 877–82.
9. Ibid., p. 882.
10. Richard Sobel, "Beyond Empathy," *Perspectives in Biology and Medicine* 51, no. 3 (2008): 471–78.
11. If we work with Sobel's definition we can see a modern psychiatric recapitulation and development of a basic insight of the economist and moral philosopher Adam Smith, who claims that empathy (he uses the term "sympathy" for this phenomenon) was a central capacity necessary for ethics. It is far from automatic, Smith insisted, and requires discipline and imagination. Adam Smith, *The Theory of Moral Sentiments*, ed.

D. D. Raphael and A. L. Macfie (Indianapolis, IN: Liberty Classics, 1982), pp. 8–23. See also the comparison between David Hume's notions of "sympathy" and those of Adam Smith in Larry R. Churchill's *Self-Interest and Universal Health Care: Why Well-Insured Americans Should Support Coverage for Everyone* (Cambridge, MA: Harvard University Press, 1994), pp. 67–72.

12. One cautionary tale about empathy. The insightful *New York Times* editorial writer David Brooks devoted a column to empathy on September 29, 2011. Writing from a posture of suspicion about the claims being made for empathy, Brooks says that American culture is currently experiencing an "empathy craze" that attributes too much to this capacity, especially when we assume it is the primary capacity for ensuring good moral choices. Brooks initially is careful to give empathy its due, citing neuroscience studies that confirm the existence of "mirror neurons" in the brain that enables this capacity. Yet his overall message is one of skepticism about how far empathy can take us, as reflected in the title to his essay, "The Limits of Empathy." Brooks finally argues not against empathy per se, but against accepting empathy as a remedy for ethical lapses. "It's insufficient," he says, and must be guided by "codes"; and in the end he dismisses empathy as a "sideshow," whereas moral codes become for the ethical person the surer "sources of identity." The reason to cite Brooks is that his column has a wide readership, and also because his dismissive critique is a conceptual misfire, best addressed not to empathy, but to what Sobel would term "sympathy." Brooks's objections are really to an unthinking and reactive emotional echoing. I know of no serious thinker who actually believes that empathy is the sum total of ethics, and we are not making that claim here. Rather our argument is that empathy is a basic or fundamental capacity, one central to both good healing skills and to ethics. Without empathy it is impossible to know how to use codes in the moral life with any skill. A richer and more accurate understanding of the cognitive and imaginative aspects of empathy, similar to that of our patient informants, would have led Brooks to write a different editorial. Perhaps we can say, in balance, that no single faculty or capacity—even empathy—can be embraced as the final answer, as all we ever need, either in ethics or in portraying the therapeutic practitioner. And this includes "codes," which are no less subject to misuse and abuse than empathic insights. Indeed, one of our main arguments in this book is that what turns out to be key in therapeutic relationships is protean, a pluralistic phenomenon, which is why we are not arguing for a theory with a hierarchy of concepts and skills, but simply seeking to put on display the range of capacities that patients tell us are helpful in this process. The elements in therapeutic relations are several, their movements are dynamic

and context specific, but follow discernible patterns. Our task here is to map these patterns but to resist the temptation to put it all together in a tight formula. David Brooks, "The Limits of Empathy," *New York Times*, September 29, 2011, p. A25.

13. Piero Ferrucci, *The Power of Kindness: The Unexpected Benefits of Leading a Compassionate Life* (New York: Penguin, 2007), p. 112.

14. See Churchill's analysis of the compassionate response of the Good Samaritan in his *Rationing Health Care in America: Perceptions and Principles of Justice* (Notre Dame, IN: University of Notre Dame Press, 1987), pp. 34–37.

15. Although widely circulated and repeated, this is likely an adaptation of another Buddhist teaching found at SN 45.2 Upaddha Sutta: Half (of the Holy Life) translated from the Pali by Thanissaro © Bhikkhu.

16. Charles G. Roland, *William Osler's The Master-Word in Medicine* (Springfield, IL: Charles C. Thomas, 1972), p. 31. This was an address that Osler gave to the medical students at the University of Toronto in 1903.

Chapter 3

1. For an excellent summary of recent thinking on multitasking and its liabilities, see Christine Rosen's "The Myth of Multitasking," *New Atlantis* 20 (Spring 2008): 105–10, http://www.thenewatlantis.com/publications/the-myth-of-multitasking, accessed on April 27, 2013 .

2. Jodi Halpern, *From Detached Concern to Empathy: Humanizing Medical Practice* (New York: Oxford University Press, 2001), pp. 59–60, 85–86. See also Rita Charon's innovative work, especially her article "Narrative Medicine: A Model for Empathy, Reflection, Profession, and Trust," *JAMA* 286, no. 15 (2001): 1897–902. The role and uses of empathy take a somewhat different turn in psychiatry. For an excellent discussion see Jennifer Radden and John Z. Sadler, *The Virtuous Psychiatrist: Character Ethics in Psychiatric Practice* (New York: Oxford University Press, 2010), pp. 26ff. and 124ff. For an excellent discussion of the importance of empathic relations in pediatrics see Margaret E. Mohrmann's *Attending Children: A Doctor's Education* (Washington, DC: Georgetown University Press, 2005).

3. Jerome Groopman, *How Doctors Think* (Boston: Houghton Mifflin, 2007).

4. See David Schenck and Larry R. Churchill, *Healers: Extraordinary Clinicians at Work* (New York: Oxford University Press, 2012), especially chapter 6, which provides details on recent research in this area and a model for how expectancy can affect outcomes.

5. Ibid., pp. 170ff.
6. Ibid., p. 15.

Chapter 4

1. In spite of attention to pain as a medical vital sign, there continue to be indications of the magnitude of the problem. The annual national economic cost to American society is estimated to be $560–635 billion. Committee on Advancing Pain Research, Care, and Education, Board on Health Sciences Policy, Institute of Medicine of the National Academies, *Relieving Pain in America: A Blueprint for Transforming Prevention, Care, Education, and Research* (Washington, DC: National Academies Press, 2011), p. 1, http://books.nap.edu/openbook.php?record_id=13172&page 1, accessed on April 27, 2013 .

2. René Descartes, *The Philosophical Works of Descartes*, vol. 1, trans. Elizabeth S. Haldane and G. R. T. Ross (Cambridge: Cambridge University Press, 1970). See especially the "Meditations on the First Philosophy," pp. 144ff. The term "Cartesian" is broadly used to indicate a large number of different approaches, all of which take as axiomatic a mind/body dichotomy. Such a mind/body split is increasingly out of favor in contemporary neuroscience. See, for example, Antonio Damasio, *The Feeling of What Happens: Body and Emotion in the Making of Consciousness* (New York: Harcourt Brace, 1999), or the more philosophically oriented work of Patricia Churchland in *Braintrust: What Neuroscience Tells Us about Morality* (Princeton: Princeton University Press, 2011).

3. See Elaine Scarry, *The Body in Pain: The Making and Unmaking of the World* (New York: Oxford University Press, 1985).

4. John Keats, *Letters*, April 21, 1819. See David Perkins, ed., *English Romantic Writers* (New York: Harcourt, Brace & World, 1967), pp. 1225–26.

5. The National Center for Complementary and Alternative Medicine reports that in 2007 more than 38 percent of adults and 12 percent of children in the United States were using CAM practitioners, and the trend was growing. See http://nccam.nih.gov/news/camstats/2007/camsurvey_fs1.htm, accessed on April 27, 2013 .

6. See David Schenck and Larry R. Churchill, *Healers: Extraordinary Clinicians at Work* (New York: Oxford University Press, 2012).

7. The integrative health model seeks to treat the person as a whole, combining conventional allopathic or "Western" medicine with complementary practices such as acupuncture or herbal medicine. Several major medical centers in the United States have robust integrative health services.

8. The full quote from Toynbee is "Death is Un-American, and an affront to every citizen's inalienable right to life, liberty and the pursuit of happiness." Clearly Toynbee was not endorsing this view, but simply reflecting what he observed about American culture. See "Changing Attitudes towards Death in the Modern Western World," in Arnold Toynbee et al., *Man's Concern with Death* (St. Louis, MO: McGraw-Hill, 1969), p. 131.

9. We single out two philosophers, although a great number could be mentioned. See Michel de Montaigne, *The Complete Essays of Montaigne*, trans. Donald M. Frame (Stanford, CA: Stanford University Press, 1958), pp. 56–68; and Martin Heidegger, *Being and Time*, trans. John Macquarrie and Edward Robinson (New York: Harper & Row, 1962), especially "Division Two: Dasein and Temporality," pp. 274–311.

10. The sources documenting end-of-life costs are numerous, but the professional practices and patient and family attitudes that produce these costs are infrequently analyzed. The *New York Times* published a report that helped to highlight both the professional and social values. See Reed Abelson, "Weighing Medical Costs of End-of-Life Care," *New York Times*, December 22, 2009, http://www.nytimes.com/2009/12/23/health/23ucla.html?pagewanted=all, accessed on April 27, 2013 .

11. Elisabeth Kübler-Ross, *On Death and Dying* (New York: Macmillan, 1969).

12. In saying there are no extended accounts of healing in the day-to-day lives of dying patients we do not mean to minimize or disregard the excellent hospice and palliative care literature focused on healing experiences of the terminally ill. Yet most of these accounts are largely practical advice for caregivers and sometimes for patients, rather than the more extended phenomenological account from the patient's point of view that we offer here. They do not follow patients over time with the motif of healing as the primary focus.

13. T. S. Eliot, "Little Gidding, Four Quartets," in *The Complete Poems and Plays, 1909–1950* (San Diego, CA: Harcourt, Brace, Jovanovich, 1971), p. 139.

14. William Wordsworth, "Ode: Intimations of Immortality from Recollections of Early Childhood," in *English Romantic Writers*, ed. David Perkins (New York: Harcourt, Brace & World, 1967), p. 281.

Chapter 5

1. This example is taken from an unused portion of a clinician interview conducted for the study on which *Healers* is based.

2. By the term "phenomenology" in the subheading for this section we indicate a method for thinking. "Doing phenomenology" hereto will mean

setting aside concepts and terms we ordinarily use to talk about patients and patient experiences. We do this in an effort to get a fresh look at what is really going on. A fresh look at the "phenomena." For a comprehensive examination of phenomenology, including summaries of the thinking of the major figures in the field, see Dermot Moran's *Introduction to Phenomenology* (London: Routledge, 2000). An excellent use of phenomenological methods in medical ethics can be found in Richard M. Zaner's *Ethics and the Clinical Encounter* (Englewood Cliffs, NJ: Prentice Hall, 1988).

3. Those who embrace "autonomy" as a primary ethical principle for patients may find this shift to shared agency troubling. We will deal with this issue in detail in chapter 6, where we discuss the adequacy of the regnant principles of contemporary bioethics more thoroughly.

4. The frequency of medical errors, especially those leading to a patient's death, is sobering. See the Institute of Medicine report *To Err Is Human: Building a Safer Health System*, ed. Linda T. Kohn, Janet M. Corrigan, and Molla S. Donaldson (Washington, DC: National Academy Press, 2000).

5. Here a long list of authors and articles could be cited. A volume that contains many of the strongest objections to a principle-based approach to bioethics is Edwin R. DuBose, Ron Hamel, and Laurence J. O'Connell, eds., *A Matter of Principles? Ferment in U.S. Bioethics* (Valley Forge, PA: Trinity Press International, 1994).

6. See David Schenck and Larry R. Churchill, "Ethics and Medicine: Healing the Wounds of Fate," in *Healers: Extraordinary Clinicians at Work* (New York: Oxford University Press, 2012), pp. 212–42.

7. One way, in fact, to define vulnerability is to speak of it as the ongoing possibility for that which is tacit in our daily lives to become focal, to demand immediate attention. This ongoing and immediate possibility of disruption—the eruption of the tacit into the focal—this is the elemental vulnerability in which we move every moment. So going out of balance is no surprise. And regaining balance is no surprise. This, in fact, is a definition of living, a definition of being.

8. Among those who have spoken of the vulnerability of patients and the acts of helping by professionals as fundamental to medical ethics the best is Edmund Pellegrino. Of special note is his article "Toward a Reconstruction of Medical Morality," *Journal of Philosophy and Medicine* 4, no. 1 (1979): 32–56. Here Pellegrino speaks of patient vulnerability as "the fact of illness," and the willingness of physicians to help as "the act of profession." This article is developed more systematically is his book with David Thomasma, *A Philosophical Basis of Medical Practice* (New York: Oxford University Press, 1981). In this latter version vulnerability is described as an "axiom" that calls into play a professional response.

9. See Erwin W. Straus, "The Upright Posture," *Psychiatric Quarterly* 26 (1952): 529–61.

10. For elaboration of the points made in this paragraph see Annemarie Mol, *The Logic of Care: Health and the Problem of Patient Choice* (London: Routledge, 2008).

Chapter 6

1. A patient-centered approach to research is the hallmark of a new federal research program, the Patient-Centered Outcomes Research Institute (PCORI), as called for in the Patient Protection and Affordable Care Act of 2010. This is a most welcome development, especially since it strongly urges the inclusion of patients and families of patients in the research teams.

2. The authors most responsible for the elevation of these three principles, and the fourth, nonmaleficence, are Tom Beauchamp and James Childress, whose work has helped to push the field of bioethics into national prominence since the appearance of the first edition of their *Principles of Biomedical Ethics* (New York: Oxford University Press) in 1979. This work is now in a seventh edition. As Larry Churchill has argued elsewhere, the major problems with a principled approach are most evident not in the work of Beauchamp and Childress, but those in the larger bioethics community who have adopted these principles and often speak and write as if this approach is the only one that matters. See Larry R. Churchill's "Rejecting Principlism, Affirming Principles," in *A Matter of Principles? Ferment in U.S. Bioethics*, ed. Edwin R. DuBose, Ron Hamel, and Laurence J. O'Connell (Valley Forge, PA: Trinity Press International, 1994), pp. 325–35. To their credit, Beauchamp and Childress have provided greater recognition for the concerns we discuss here in each successive edition of their work. The seventh edition of *Principles of Biomedical Ethics* includes a good discussion of virtues under a chapter entitled "Moral Character," pp.30–61. They might well agree with our overall emphasis here, if not all the particulars of our arguments. See, for example, from the seventh edition of *Principles*: "What often matters most in the moral life is not adherence to moral rules, but having a reliable character, a good moral sense, and an appropriate emotional responsiveness." p. 30. Or consider this statement: "Those physicians and nurses who express no compassion in their behavior fail to provide what patients need most." p. 38.

For a distinctive but complementary critique of exclusive reliance on principles in bioethics see Larry R. Churchill and David Schenck, "One Cheer for Bioethics: Engaging the Moral Experiences of Patients and

Practitioners beyond the Big Decisions," *Cambridge Quarterly of Healthcare Ethics* 14 (2005): 389–403. See also the insightful work of Howard Brody, *The Healer's Power* (New Haven, CT: Yale University Press, 1992), where he argues at length for a broadening of medical ethics beyond principles to include a virtuous use of power, and a sharing of power with patients. Brody's model of "shared power" is very compatible with our work here. The chief difference is that our notion of "doubled-agency" begins from patients' felt need for an augmented power to deal with their illnesses, and a subsequent granting of that power to clinicians. By contrast, "shared power" suggests a contribution by the patient to a power otherwise presumptively held by the professional. Hence there are different beginning points and different assumptions about whose perspective is assumed to be at the center. Our interviews are extended testimony to why this difference in starting points and assumptions is morally important. We will underline these differences in our reformulations and as we look at bioethics as a field, medical ethics codes, and the moral agenda of medical education.

Much of our analysis is also quite compatible with feminist ethics and feminist bioethics, especially the various feminist emphases on "caring," focusing on routine relationships as morally important, and the consequent insistence by many feminist writers on a less-formal, less-principled process for understanding the basics of healthcare relationships. The best of feminist writings as they relate to our current thesis are those of Margaret Urban Walker. Walker's description of the dominant "theoretical-juridical model" of morality and her critique of its shortcomings is one of most trenchant reformulations within the feminist tradition, and one very relevant to our overall thesis in this book. She is especially critical of the modeling of authority, epistemology, and science that informs the theoretical-juridical paradigm, and she calls for an "expressive-collaborative model" that embodies a more "descriptively rich and politically critical" approach to ethics. See especially Walker's *Moral Understandings*, 2nd ed. (New York: Oxford University Press, 2007), pp. 30ff, 55ff).

Finally, a characteristically prescient reinterpretation of principles in bioethics and medical ethics was undertaken in a review article by Arthur W. Frank in *The Hastings Center Report*, July–August 1998, pp. 37–41. Drawing upon the work of Paul A. Komesaroff and his notion of "microethics," Frank finds three principles of importance in the patient narratives he reviews. These are: (1) *representation* of self and others; (2) *reciprocity* between the sick and the well; and (3) *reconciliation* with the illness, with oneself, and with others. These all function, Frank argues, within the larger context of awareness of the contingency of one's life. Frank argues that foregrounding relationships—as his principles clearly do—would require health professionals to think and behave very differently. Frank calls this "the beginnings of a yet-unarticulated ethic" (p. 37). The articulation of this as-yet-unspoken ethics is a good description of the task we have undertaken in this book. See also Komesaroff's article "From Bioethics to Microethics: Ethical Debate and Clinical Medicine," in *Troubled Bodies: Critical Perspectives on Postmodernism, Medical Ethics and the Body*, ed. Paul A. Komesaroff (Durham, NC: Duke University Press, 1995).

A recent study seeking to understand if and when the standard bioethics principles are used concluded that while the subjects in the study espoused these principles, the situational factors of the cases they were presented were of greater importance; hence their decisions were better described as casuistic in nature. See Katie Page, "The Four Principles: Can They Be Measured and Do They Predict Ethical Decision Making?" *BMC Medical Ethics* 13, no. 10 (2012), http://www.biomedcentral.com/1472–6939/13/10, accessed on April 27, 2013 .

3. See Peter Gay's classic account of the centrality of politics, with physics as the core paradigm, in *The Enlightenment: An Interpretation, vol. 2: The Science of Freedom* (New York: W. W. Norton, 1969), especially "The Science of Man," pp. 167–215.

4. To be helpful, normative accounts should attend closely to the norms implicit in the daily practice. Whether these practices and norms actually achieve the intended good depends on the judgments of stakeholders, most prominently, providers *and* patients. The claims on offer here are that bioethics and its principles have largely failed (1) to pay close enough attention to the relationships that constitute daily practice, and (2) to give proper due to patients' experiences of health care. Bioethicists susceptible to these claims are like basketball analysts who comment only on rules and referees. They become preoccupied with steps out of bounds and fouls, but fail to address the complex ball movements and offensive and defensive patterns within the routine field of play.

5. It should be noted that we have experienced this more in the expectations and habits of younger clinicians, who have grown to maturity in an era of autonomy, than for their older colleagues, who were largely still nurtured in professional norms of beneficent paternalism.

6. For a detailed discussion of the origins and values of "beneficence" as a principle, see Larry R. Churchill's entry in the *Encyclopedia of Bioethics*, 4th ed., ed. Bruce Jennings (New York: Gale-Macmillan, 2013), forthcoming.

7. A final comment about the hazards of autonomy is in order here as it relates especially to the U.S. context. As Michael Sandel has recently argued, the United States has moved from being a market economy to being a market society (*What Money Can't Buy: The Moral Limits of Markets*

[New York: Farrar, Straus and Giroux, 2012]). This is clearly the case for how we understand and value healthcare services. One of the implications of this dominance of market thinking is the way it tends to turn respect for autonomy as a political concept into respect for consumer autonomy in freely choosing from a range of services. In this shift, weighing choices for their fit with one's life values turns into a valuing of the capacity for savvy shopping for goods and services. Instead of the patient-as-person, we have the patient-as-consumer. There are many facets of American culture that endorse and encourage just this shift in the ethics of health care. Our aim here is not an extended argument against this shift, but rather simply to point attention to this additional hazard embedded in the typical bioethical modeling of healthcare ethics. It might be thought that professional ethics will provide protection against this commercialization of health care and healthcare interactions. Indeed, the whole idea of a professional ethics is to provide an independent metric for judging things like market forces, patient demands, or political intrusions into care. Why medical ethics has been only partially effective in that protective role is because it too has become commercialized and isolated from patient experiences by its self-protective and trade-union agendas.

8. At this point the skeptic might object that what we have portrayed here is an idealized form of patient-clinician relationships that existed only in the past, perhaps even in an idealized past. In the current healthcare environment that values efficiency on an industrial model, what we have described is frequently impossible, or at best highly truncated. The skeptic will likely further note that most of our examples come from chronic disease care and not from the more procedurally oriented practices, where high volume or through-put is the chief norm. Is this really a viable model for healthcare relationships that occurs so often between strangers? Even if it is desirable, who actually has time for developing the kind of relationships we describe here?

Our response to such skepticism is as follows. First we reject the assumption that what we propose here as ideal always takes more time. As the clinicians described in *Healers* repeatedly pointed out, the most desirable relational skills are not extra things to do, not a new checklist, but are ways of doing differently what already must be done. Presenting oneself as a clinician who is trustworthy is usually not a matter of additional clock time, but being truly present for the time one does have—making a connection, showing interest in the person behind the disease, and assuming a demeanor of caring and continued availability. There is also a growing body of evidence that what we present here results in better patient outcomes, and increased job satisfaction for clinicians. It is in fact a major deficit of the regnant model of "good" health care that it does not give a more prominent place to the relational dimensions. Finally, we would invite the skeptic to reread chapter 3 and note that the failures described there were typically marked by inefficiency, poor outcomes, lack of continuity, and ultimately increased cost burdens to clinicians, patients, and society.

9. http://www.ama-assn.org/ama/pub/physician-resources/medical-ethics/code-medical-ethics/principles-medical-ethics.page?, accessed on June 25, 2012.

10. Ludwig Edelstein, *The Hippocratic Oath: Text, Translation and Interpretation*, supplement to the *Bulletin of the History of Medicine*, no. 1 (Baltimore, MD: Johns Hopkins Press, 1943).

11. AMA Code of Medical Ethics.

12. "American College of Physicians Ethics Manual, Sixth Edition," in *Annals of Internal Medicine* 156, no. 1 (pt. 2, Supplement, 2012): 73–104. There is no indication, even in this very thoughtful manual, of serious patient input into its key ideas.

13. See David Mechanic, "Changing Medical Organization and the Erosion of Trust," *Milbank Quarterly* 74 (1996): 171–89. Also, sociologist William Sullivan has written eloquently on this point of the need for physicians to look to the public welfare and patients' good to regain their lost professionalism.

14. See the Code of Ethics for Nurses with Interpretive Statements at http://www.nursingworld.org/MainMenuCategories/EthicsStandards/CodeofEthicsforNurses/Code-of-Ethics.pdf, accessed on June 25, 2012.

15. Ibid.

16. Sarah Breier-Mackie, "Medical Ethics and Nursing Ethics: Is There Really Any Difference?" *Gastroenterology Nursing* 29, no. 2 (March–April 2006): 182–83.

17. Vanderbilt University Medical Center's list of Patient Rights and Responsibilities is a typical example. See http://www.mc.vanderbilt.edu/documents/main/files/PatientRightsResponsibilities07.pdf, accessed on April 27, 2013 . We did not do a systematic survey, but the Johns Hopkins University Hospital, Duke University Hospital, and Massachusetts General Hospital lists of patient rights and responsibilities are almost identical to Vanderbilt's.

18. Almost two decades ago the Pew-Fetzer Task Force recommended a paradigm for health care they called "relationship-centered care." We largely concur with their aims but add a cautionary note. "Relationship-centered care" will be no better than conventional medical care if professionals are defining the relationship in isolation from, or with disregard for, the experiences of patients. Relationships are highly important precisely because they teach clinicians how to focus on, and finally help, the patient. Every

effort to reformulate healthcare ethics will be suspect unless it puts the patient's understandings of their healthcare needs clearly in the center. When the patient is truly central in this way appropriate relationships will follow. See Carol P. Tresolini and the Pew-Fetzer Task Force, *Health Professions Education and Relationship-Centered Care* (San Francisco: Pew Health Professions Commission, 1994).

19. Iris Murdoch, *The Sovereignty of Good* (London: Routledge & Kegan Paul, 1970), p. 37.
20. Ibid.

INDEX